renewing our voice

Code of Good Practice
for NGOs Responding to HIV/AIDS

Published by The NGO HIV/AIDS Code of Practice Project
Copyright © The NGO HIV/AIDS Code of Practice Project, 2004
PO Box 372, chemin des Crets, 1211 Geneva 19, Switzerland
Telephone: +41 22 730 42 22
Fax: +41 22 733 03 95
Web: www.ifrc.org/what/health/hivaids/code/

The NGO HIV/AIDS Code of Practice Project is a joint initiative of:

- ActionAid International
- CARE USA
- Global Health Council
- Global Network of People Living with HIV/AIDS (GNP+)
- Grupo Pela Vidda
- Hong Kong AIDS Foundation
- International Council of AIDS Service Organisations (ICASO)
- International Federation of Red Cross and Red Crescent Societies
- International Harm Reduction Association
- International HIV/AIDS Alliance
- World Council of Churches

Author: Julia Cabassi
Editor: David Wilson

First draft version: March 2004
First final edition: December 2004

ISBN 0 85598 553 4

A catalogue record for this publication is available from The British Library and the US Library of
Congress.

Distributed for The NGO HIV/AIDS Code of Practice Project worldwide by Oxfam GB.

Available from Oxfam Publishing, 274 Banbury Road, Oxford, OX2 7DZ, UK.
Tel: +44 (0) 1865 311311 Fax: +44 1865 312600 email: publish@oxfam.org.uk Web:
www.oxfam.org.uk/publications and from its agents and representatives throughout the world. Oxfam
GB is a registered charity, no 202918, and is a member of Oxfam International.

Renewing Our Voice: Code of Good Practice for NGOs Responding to HIV/AIDS is also available on the website
of the International Federation of Red Cross and Red Crescent Societies, with hyperlinks to secondary
source material. www.ifrc.org/what/health/hivaids/code/

The diagrams on pages 25 and 61 are from Mainstreaming HIV/AIDS in Development and
Humanitarian Programmes by Sue Holden, published by Oxfam GB, 2004, and are reproduced with the
permission of Oxfam GB.

Cover and poster designed by: Laura Amiet
Text design by: Jean-Charles Chamois
Layout by: Marie-Christine Dupont
Printed by: Imprimerie Corbaz, Montreux, Switzerland

renewing our **voice**

Code of Good Practice
for NGOs Responding to HIV/AIDS

guiding principles

organisational principles

- Involvement of PLHA and affected communities
- Multi-sectoral partnerships
- Governance
- Organisational mission and management
- Programme planning, monitoring and evaluation
- Access and equity
- Advocacy
- Research
- Scaling up

programming principles

HIV/AIDS Programming

- Cross cutting issues
- Voluntary counselling and testing (VCT)
- HIV prevention
- Treatment, care and support
- Addressing stigma and discrimination

Mainstreaming HIV/AIDS:
development and humanitarian
programming

Contents

Contents

Code signatories

Accion Ciudadana Contre el SIDA (ACCSI), Venezuela
www.internet.ve/accsi

Acción Contra el Hambre, Spain
www.accioncontraelhambre.org

ACT International
www.act-intl.org

Action Against Hunger, UK
www.aahuk.org

ActionAid International
www.actionaid.org

AfriCASO (African Council of AIDS Service Organizations)
www.africaso.net

AIDS Action Europe (AAE)

AIDS Calgary
www.aidscalgary.org

Anti-AIDS Centre, Russia

AIDS Hilfe, Austria
www.aids.at

AIDS Infoshare, Russia

AIDS Network Development Foundation (AIDSNet), Thailand

AIDS Saint John, Canada

AIDS Society of Kamloops, Canada
www.aidskamloops.bc.ca

Alan Guttmacher Institute, USA
www.agi-usa.org

Alberta Community Council on HIV, Canada

All-Ukrainian Network of PLWH

Alliance National Contre le SIDA (ANCS), Sénégal

Amnesty for Women, Germany
www.amnestyforwomen.de

AMREF (African Medical and Research Foundation) www.amref.org

APCASO (Asia Pacific Council of AIDS Service Organizations)
www.apcaso.org

APN+ (Asia-Pacific Network of People Living With HIV/AIDS)
www.gnpplus.net/regions/asiapac.html

Asociación Costarricense de Personas Viviendo con VIH/SIDA (ASO VIH/SIDA), Costa Rica

Asociación Dominicana Pro-Bienestar de la Familia (PROFAMILIA), Dominican Republic
www.profamilia.org.do

Association Marocaine de Solidarité et de Développement (AMSED), Morocco

Association Rwandaise pour le Bien-Etre Familial (ARBEF), Rwanda

Australian Federation of AIDS Organisations (AFAO)
www.afao.org

Australian Red Cross
www.redcross.org.au

British Columbia Persons with AIDS Society, Canada

Brot fur die Welt (Bread for the World)
www.brot-fuer-die-welt.org

Cameroon National Association for Family Welfare

Canada – Africa Community Health Alliance

Canadian AIDS Treatment Information Exchange (CATIE),
www.catie.ca

Canadian HIV/AIDS Legal Network
www.aidslaw.ca

Canadian Society for International Health
www.csih.org

Care International
www.care-international.org

Caribbean Regional Network for People Living with HIV/AIDS (CRN+)

Catholic Medical Mission Board, USA
www.cmmb.org

CAUSE, Canada
www.cause.ca

CEEHRN (Central and Eastern European Harm Reduction Network)
www.ceehrn.lt

Chi Heng Foundation
www.chihengfoundation.com

China Family Planning Association
www.chinafpa.org.cn

Christian Aid
www.christian-aid.org.uk

Christian Children's Fund
www.christianchildrensfund.org

Church of Sweden
www.svenskakyrkan.se

Coalition of HIV/AIDS Service Organisations, Ukraine

Community Action Resource (CARe), Trinidad

Concern Worldwide
www.concern.net

Conference of European Churches
www.cec-kek.org

Corporacion Kimirina, Ecuador

Dan Church Aid
www.dca.dk

Danish Red Cross
http://www1.drk.dk

Deutsche AIDS Hilfe e. V, Germany
www.aidshilfe.de

Diakonie Emergency Aid,
www.diakonie-katastrophenhilfe.de

DIFAM, German Institute for Medical Mission
www.difam.de

Ecumenical Advocacy Alliance
www.e-alliance.ch

Ecumenical Coalition on Tourism
www.ecotonline.org

Ecumenical Pharmaceutical Network
www.epnnetwork.org

European AIDS Treatment Group (EATG)
www.eatg.org

European Coalition for Just and Effective Drug Policies
www.encod.org

Family Planning Association of Estonia
www.amor.ee

Family Planning Association of India
www.fpaindia.com

Family Planning Association of Kenya

Family Planning Association of Malawi

Family Planning Association of Nepal
www.fpan.org

Family Planning Organization of the Philippines
www.fpop.org.ph

Federation of Family Planning Associations, Malaysia (FFPAM)
www.ffpam.org.my

Fondazione Villa Maraini, Italy
www.villamaraini.it

Global Chinese AIDS Network
www.aids.org.hk

GNP+ (Global Network of People Living with HIV/AIDS)
www.gnpplus.net

GNP+ Europe

GNP+ North America
www.gnpna.ca

GOAL
www.goal.ie

Grupo Pela Vidda, Brazil
www.pelavidda.org.br

Groupe Chrétien Contre le SIDA au Togo (GCCST)
http://membres.lycos.fr/gccst/

Healthlink Worldwide
www.healthlink.org.uk

HelpAge International
www.helpage.org

HIV/AIDS and STD Alliance, Bangladesh

Hoffnung fur Osteuropa (Hope for Eastern Europe)
www.hoffnung-fuer-osteuropa.de

Hong Kong AIDS Foundation
www.aids.org.hk

ICASO (International Council of AIDS Service Organizations)
www.icaso.org

ICW (International Community of Women Living with HIV/AIDS)
www.icw.org

Indonesian Planned Parenthood Association
www.pkbi.or.id

Initiative Privée et Communautaire de Lutte Contre Le VIH/SIDA au Burkina Faso (IPC/BF)

Inppares, Peru
www.inppares.org.pe

Interact Worldwide
www.interactworldwide.org

Interagency Coalition on AIDS and Development
www.icad-cisd.com

International Federation of Red Cross and Red Crescent Societies
www.ifrc.org

International Harm Reduction Association
www.ihra.net

International HIV/AIDS Alliance including International HIV/AIDS Alliance Madagascar, Mozambique, Ukraine, Zambia, India HIV/AIDS Alliance, Caribbean Regional Programme, China Programme, Myanmar Programme
www.aidsalliance.org

International HIV/AIDS Institute, Ukraine

International Planned Parenthood Federation (IPPF) including Central Office London, European, South Asia, Africa and Western Hemisphere regional offices)
www.ippf.org

International Planned Parenthood Federation, Laos

International Relief Teams
www.irteams.org

International Service for Human Rights
www.ishr.ch

Irish Red Cross
www.redcross.ie

Jamaica Family Planning Association

Japan AIDS & Society Association

Kazakhstan Crisis Centres Union

Kenya AIDS NGO Consortium (KANCO)
www.kanco.org

Kiribati Family Health Association

LACCASO (Latin America and Caribbean Council of AIDS Service Organizations)
www.laccaso.org

LEPRA Society, India
www.lepraindia.org

LET (NGO Life Quality Improvement Organisation) Croatia

Lutheran World Federation
www.lutheranworld.org

Lutheran World Relief
www.lwr.org

Marie Stopes Clinic Society, Bangladesh
www.mariestopes.org.uk/ww/bangladesh.htm

Marie Stopes International
www.mariestopes.org.uk

Megapolis Saratov Oblast Nongovernmental Foundation, Russia

Mexfam, Mexico
www.mexfam.org.mx

MSM: No Political Agenda
www.msmnpa.org

NACASO (North American Council of AIDS Service Organizations)

National AIDS Foundation, Mongolia
www.naf.org.mn

National AIDS Trust, UK
www.nat.org.uk

National Association of People Living with HIV/AIDS (NAPWA), Australia
www.napwa.org.au

Namibia Red Cross

Naz Foundation International
www.nfi.net

NELA (Network on Ethics, Law, HIV/AIDS, Prevention, Support & Care), Nigeria

New Way (Center of Psychosocial Information and Counseling), Georgia

Northern AIDS Connection, Canada
http://nacsns.tripod.com

Norwegian Church Aid
www.nca.no

Norwegian Red Cross
www.redcross.no

ODYSEUS, Slovak republic
www.ozodyseus.sk

OSDUY (Organization for Social
Development of Unemployed Youth),
Bangladesh

Oxfam International
www.oxfam.org

Palmyrah Workers' Development Society, India
www.pwds.org

Pathfinder International
www.pathfind.org

PLANeS, Fondation suisse pour la santé
sexuelle et reproductive
www.plan-s.ch

Plan USA
www.planusa.org

Planned Parenthood Association of South
Africa
www.ppasa.org.za

Planned Parenthood Association of Thailand
(PPAT)

Planned Parenthood Federation of America
www.plannedparenthood.org

Planned Parenthood Federation of Canada
www.ppfc.ca

Population Action International
www.populationaction.org

Population Services and Training Center
(PSTC), Bangladesh

Radda MCH-FP Centre, Bangladesh

REDLA+ (Latin American Network of
PLWHA)
www.redla.org

Regional Public Foundation - Novoye Vremya
(New Time), Russia

Reproductive Health Association of Cambodia

Roses and Rosemary, USA

Russian Association Family Planning
www.family-planning.ru

Save the Children, Canada
www.savethechildren.ca

Sensoa International
www.sensoa.be

Singapore Planned Parenthood Association
www.sppa.org.sg

Soroptimist International
www.soroptimistinternational.org

Southern African AIDS Trust (SAT)
www.satregional.org

STI/AIDS Network, Bangladesh

TAMPEP International Foundation,
www.europap.net/links/tampep.htm

Tonga Family Health Association

Tuvalu Family Health Association

UK Coalition of People Living with HIV and
AIDS (UKC)
www.ukcoalition.org

Vasavya Mahila Mandali
www.vasavya.com

Voronezh Regional Fund to Support Youth
Entrepreneurship, Russia

VSO
www.vso.org.uk

Wild Foundation
www.wild.org

Wilderness Foundation, South Africa
www.wild.org/southern_africa/wf.html

World Alliance of Reformed Churches
www.warc.ch

World Alliance of YMCAs
www.ymca.int

World Council of Churches (WCC)
www.wcc-coe.org

World Student Christian Federation
www.servingthetruth.org

World YWCA
www.worldywca.org

Executive Summary

This Code sets out a number of **Guiding Principles** (in **Chapter 2**), which apply a human rights approach to the range of HIV/AIDS-specific health, development and humanitarian work undertaken by NGOs responding to HIV/AIDS. These principles provide a common framework applicable to all NGOs engaged in responding to HIV/AIDS, and are embodied within good practice principles, which guide both how we work as NGOs (**Chapter 3 – Organisational Principles**) and what we do (**Chapter 4 – Programming Principles**). **Chapter 5** includes **Key resources** such as tool kits and manuals that can assist in putting the principles into practice. It also includes information about the process of 'signing on' to the Code and about implementation of the Code.

Guiding principles

- We advocate for the meaningful involvement of PLHA and affected communities in all aspects of the HIV/AIDS response.
- We protect and promote human rights in our work.
- We apply public health principles within our work.
- We address the causes of vulnerability to HIV infection and the impacts of HIV/AIDS.
- Our programmes are informed by evidence in order to respond to the needs of those most vulnerable to HIV/AIDS and its consequences.

Organisational principles

Chapter 3 provides good practice principles to guide how we do our work.

Involvement of PLHA and affected communities

- We foster active and meaningful involvement of PLHA and affected communities in our work.

Multi-sectoral partnerships

- We build and sustain partnerships to support coordinated and comprehensive responses to HIV/AIDS.

Governance

- We have transparent governance and are accountable to our communities/constituencies.

Organisational mission and management

- We have a clear mission, supported by strategic objectives that are achieved through good management.
- We value, support and effectively manage our human resources.
- We develop and maintain the organisational capacity necessary to support effective responses to HIV/AIDS.
- We manage financial resources in an efficient, transparent and accountable manner.

Programme planning, monitoring and evaluation

- We select appropriate partners in a transparent manner.
- We plan, monitor and evaluate programmes for effectiveness and in response to community need.

Access and equity

- Our programmes are non-discriminatory, accessible and equitable.

Advocacy

- We advocate for an enabling environment that protects and promotes the rights of PLHA and affected communities and supports effective programming.
- We plan, monitor and evaluate advocacy efforts for effectiveness and in response to community need.

Research

- We undertake and/or advocate for adequate and appropriate research to ensure responses to HIV/AIDS are informed by evidence.

Scaling up

- We work to scale up appropriate programmes while ensuring their quality and sustainability.
- We develop and maintain community ownership and organisational capacity to support scaling up of programmes.
- We monitor and evaluate programmes that are scaled up.

Programming principles

Chapter 4 provides good practice principles to guide:

- HIV/AIDS programming, including HIV prevention; voluntary testing and counselling; treatment, care and support; and addressing stigma and discrimination; and
- mainstreaming HIV/AIDS within development and humanitarian programmes.

The principles in Chapter 4 relate to services, programmes and advocacy work (the term 'programmes' is used to encompass all three). Given the wide diversity of programming work undertaken by NGOs, different good practice principles will be applicable to different organisations.

HIV/AIDS Programming

Cross cutting issues

- Our HIV/AIDS programmes are integrated to reach and meet the diverse needs of PLHA and affected communities.
- Our HIV/AIDS programmes raise awareness and build the capacity of communities to respond to HIV/AIDS.
- We advocate for an enabling environment that protects and promotes the rights of PLHA and affected communities and supports effective HIV/AIDS programmes.

Voluntary Counselling and Testing (VCT)

- We provide and/or advocate for voluntary counselling and testing services that are accessible and confidential.

HIV prevention

- We provide and/or advocate for comprehensive HIV prevention programmes to meet the variety of needs of individuals and communities.
- Our HIV prevention programmes enable individuals to develop the skills to protect themselves and/or others from HIV infection.
- Our HIV prevention programmes ensure that individuals have access to and information about the use of commodities to prevent HIV infection.
- We provide and/or advocate for comprehensive harm reduction programmes for people who inject drugs.

Treatment, care and support

- We provide and/or advocate for comprehensive treatment, care and support programmes.
- We enable PLHA and affected communities to meet their treatment, care and support needs.

Addressing stigma and discrimination

- We enable PLHA and affected communities to understand their rights and respond to discrimination and its consequences.
- We monitor and respond to systemic discrimination.
- We enable communities to understand and address HIV/AIDS-related stigma.
- We foster partnerships with human rights institutions, legal services and unions to promote and protect the human rights of PLHA and affected communities.

Mainstreaming HIV/AIDS: development and humanitarian programming

- We review our development and humanitarian programmes to assess their relevance to reducing vulnerability to HIV infection and addressing the consequences of HIV/AIDS.
- We work in partnerships to maximise the access of PLHA and affected communities to an integrated range of programmes to meet their needs.
- We design or adapt development programmes to reduce vulnerability to HIV infection and meet the needs of PLHA and affected communities.
- We ensure that our humanitarian programmes reduce vulnerability to HIV infection and address the needs of PLHA and affected communities.
- Our programmes for orphans and vulnerable children affected by HIV/AIDS (OVC) are child-centred, family- and community-focused and rights-based.
- We advocate for an environment that supports effective mainstreaming of HIV/AIDS.
- We advocate for an enabling environment that addresses the underlying causes of vulnerability to HIV/AIDS.

Introduction

1.1 Context

HIV/AIDS is an unprecedented global development challenge, and one that has already caused too much hardship, illness and death. To date, the epidemic has claimed the lives of 20 million people, and over 37 million worldwide are now living with HIV/AIDS.[1] In 2003, almost 5 million people became newly infected with HIV, the greatest number in any one year since the beginning of the epidemic.[2] AIDS is a crisis that is extraordinary in its scale. To stand any chance of effectively responding to the epidemic, we have to treat it both as an emergency and as a long-term development issue.[3]

Social, cultural, economic and legal factors exacerbate the spread of HIV and heighten the impact of HIV/AIDS. In almost all cases, poor and socially marginalised people are disproportionately vulnerable to HIV/AIDS and its consequences. The UN Millennium Declaration, and the goals it sets, highlight the interconnectedness between development goals and the need to address the causes of vulnerability to HIV/AIDS and its impacts, by alleviating poverty through sustainable development, the promotion of gender equality and access to education.[4] The overwhelming burden of the epidemic is borne by developing countries, where the vast majority of the people most affected by, and vulnerable to, HIV/AIDS do not have access to even a basic set of HIV prevention, treatment, care and support services and programmes.[5]

1.2 Building on the global momentum

In recent years there has been growing momentum to address the global HIV/AIDS crisis, more so than at any other time in the course of the pandemic. The United Nations General Assembly Special Session on HIV/AIDS (UNGASS), held in June 2001, resulted in the unanimous adoption by member states of the Declaration of Commitment on HIV/AIDS that set time-bound targets against which governments and the UN itself may be held accountable.[6,7] Non-government organisations (NGOs) are playing a critical role in advocating, at both national and international levels, for governments, UN agencies and others to take concrete action to make these commitments a reality.[8]

CHAPTER 1

Financial resources are being more effectively mobilised in an effort to scale up proven strategies to address HIV/AIDS. Spending on HIV/AIDS in low- and middle-income countries increased from $1 billion in 2000 to $3.9 billion in 2002 and a projected $6.1 billion in 2004.[9] While this falls far short of the estimated $12 billion needed by 2005, the progress made in resource mobilisation is encouraging.[10]

However, the life-saving benefits of antiretroviral (ARV) therapy have been experienced predominantly in industrialised countries, while millions of people in developing countries continue to die each year. Between 5 and 6 million people in developing counties urgently need access to ARVs.[11] NGOs have played a significant role in highlighting this fundamental inequity, bringing pressure to bear on governments, the UN system and pharmaceutical companies. While there are significant challenges in providing ARVs to large numbers of people in resource-limited settings, significant steps are now being taken in this direction. Drug prices have fallen in recent years, particularly in the wake of increased generic competition in the pharmaceutical sector. WHO and UNAIDS have launched a global initiative, 'Three by Five', which aims to provide ARV therapy to 3 million people with HIV/AIDS in developing countries by the end of 2005.[12]

1.3 Applying lessons learned to scaling up

Over the past 20 years, research and practice have generated an impressive body of knowledge about how to respond effectively to HIV/AIDS. While learning will continue, we must harness the current momentum. We must use what we already know to guide the allocation of resources and develop and sustain responses of sufficient scale to affect the dynamics of the epidemic (see section 3.10 Scaling up). We must concentrate our resources where they will make the most difference in slowing the spread of the epidemic and meeting the needs of people living with HIV/AIDS (PLHA) and affected communities. This requires HIV/AIDS-specific responses and the integration of HIV/AIDS within broader health programming, including sexual and reproductive health. It also requires HIV/AIDS to be mainstreamed within development and humanitarian programming to address the underlying causes of vulnerability to HIV infection and the complex consequences of HIV/AIDS.

The diverse range of NGOs now responding to HIV/AIDS – including development, humanitarian, sexual and reproductive health and human rights, as well as specialist HIV/AIDS NGOs – have a wealth of expertise and capacity that must be effectively tapped, resourced and coordinated in order to bring to scale the range of responses needed to have an effect on the course of the pandemic. This Code draws on the knowledge and experience gained over the past

20 years, documenting evidence-informed good practice principles to strengthen the work of the many different types of NGO now involved in the response.

1.4 Accountability and independence of NGOs

What do we mean by 'NGO'?

For convenience, we use the term NGO to encompass the wide range of organisations that can be characterised as 'not for profit' and 'non-government'. This includes Community-Based Organisations (CBOs), Faith-Based Organisations (FBOs) and organisations of affected communities, including people living with HIV/AIDS, sex workers and women's groups, among many others, who are active in the HIV/AIDS response (see also section 1.6 Who the Code is for).

What do we mean by 'affected communities'?

The term is used to encompass the range of people affected by HIV/AIDS – people at particular risk of HIV infection and those who bear a disproportionate burden of the impact of HIV/AIDS. This varies from country to country, depending on the nature of the epidemic concerned (see also section 2.5 Cross-cutting issues: addressing population vulnerability).

Communities must be an integral part of what NGOs are and what we do. A genuine commitment to the involvement of PLHA and affected communities in responding to HIV/AIDS is not simply the expression of a commitment to ensure that communities have control over their own health. Rather, it acknowledges that the experience of individuals and communities is an essential ingredient in effective community response to the challenges of HIV/AIDS. It is at the level of individuals and communities that HIV infection occurs and the impacts of HIV/AIDS are felt. It is communities themselves that take up the challenges posed by HIV/AIDS and work to find appropriate solutions. When efforts to respond to HIV/AIDS are grounded in the lived experiences of those affected, they are far more likely to address the many factors that shape HIV risk, HIV transmission and the experience of living with HIV/AIDS.

NGOs take an active role in advocating for the accountability of governments, private and public sector agencies and others. We too must be accountable to the communities we are part of, work with, represent and serve. Accountability, transparency and effective stewardship of resources are crucial. This is vital to our credibility, both with the communities we work with and with the agencies that provide the necessary resources for our work. Accountability to, and a demonstrated involvement of, communities strengthens the legitimacy of our advocacy voice. This imperative is further highlighted as more resources become available. We need to ensure that donors do not influence our priorities in ways that are inconsistent with our stated missions and goals. We must protect and maintain the right to independently determine our own priorities in line with the needs and aspirations of the communities we serve.

1.5 Fostering partnerships

In every country, the complexities of HIV/AIDS exceed the capability of any single sector. The pandemic demands mobilisation and collaboration at community, national and international levels. It requires HIV-specific responses and responses that address the causes of vulnerability to HIV/AIDS and its impacts. It also requires greater coherence, coordination and consistency between sectors.[13] Multi-sectoral partnerships are essential for an effective response. Government, civil society (including NGOs) and the private and public sectors must all play their part. We need to ensure that we complement each other's strategies and actively collaborate, while respecting each other's independence and acknowledging differences. Transparency, critical thinking, learning and sharing are essential elements of successful partnerships.

1.6 About the Code

What the Code is for

The Code provides a shared vision of principles for good practice in our programming and advocacy that can guide our work, and to which we can commit and be held accountable.

Since the mid- to late 1990s, there has been a considerable increase in the number and range of NGOs involved in responding to the multiple challenges presented by HIV/AIDS: NGOs undertaking HIV/AIDS work; NGOs integrating HIV/AIDS-specific interventions within other health programming, such as sexual and reproductive health and child and maternal health programmes; and NGOs mainstreaming HIV/AIDS within development, human rights and humanitarian programming. There have also been significant changes in the global funding environment, particularly in ensuring that the lessons learned over the past 20 years are used to guide the allocation of resources in scaling up responses to HIV/AIDS.

These changes both support and complicate the process of expanding the scale and impact of NGO programmes, which is so urgently needed. The proliferation of NGOs and programmes has, at times, occurred at the expense of accountability and quality programming, and has led to fragmentation of the NGO 'voice' in the HIV/AIDS response. The purpose of the Code is to address these new challenges by:

- outlining and building wider commitment to principles and practices, informed by evidence, that underscore successful NGO responses to HIV/AIDS
- assisting 'Supporting NGOs' to improve the quality and cohesiveness of our work and our accountability to our partners and beneficiary communities
- fostering greater collaboration between the variety of 'Supporting NGOs' now actively engaged in responding to the HIV/AIDS pandemic, and
- renewing the 'voice' of NGOs responding to HIV/AIDS by enabling us to commit to a shared vision of good practice in our programming and advocacy.

The Code of Good Practice provides guidance to Supporting NGOs in their work with their NGO partners (see below, Who the code is for). The principles set out in the Code can be used to guide:

- organisational planning
- the development, implementation and evaluation of programmes, including advocacy programmes
- advocacy efforts to ensure effective scaling-up of our responses to HIV/AIDS
- allocation of resources based on the principles it outlines, and
- advocacy efforts to ensure that the essential range of programmes is available where they are needed.

What the Code is not

Given the diversity of epidemics around the world, the Code is not intended to be a detailed practice manual. This would be a far larger task, and would be extremely difficult to achieve in a manner appropriate to all the different types of epidemic. It does, however, outline the main population groups that are vulnerable in different contexts (see section 2.5 Cross-cutting issues: addressing population vulnerability). It is envisaged that signatory NGOs will apply the Code in different ways, such as developing training modules with partner NGOs or member organisations, or using the principles it contains to develop indicators appropriate for the context in which they work, which can then be used when developing, implementing and evaluating specific programmes. The value of the Code will depend upon how these principles are applied by signatory NGOs over time, in line with the nature of each country's epidemic and context.

Who the Code is for

'Supporting NGOs'

The scale and complexity of the global pandemic mean that there are large numbers and a great diversity of NGOs working in HIV/AIDS. The Code addresses this diverse range of NGOs – including those engaged in HIV/AIDS, development, humanitarian, sexual and reproductive health, and human rights work. In particular, it is written for and designed to assist NGOs that provide other NGOs implementing programmes in-country with any of the following: technical support; financial support; capacity development and/or advocacy support.

We refer to this target audience as 'Supporting NGOs', and they are likely to be national or international NGOs.

Many of the principles set out in the Code can be applied to the work of Supporting NGOs with their NGO partners in-country. Partner NGOs can use the Code to hold signatory Supporting NGOs, with whom they work, accountable, while both types of NGO can use the Code as a common tool in guiding their collaborative work.

Any NGO that supports the aims of the Code

The Code can also be used to support the work of any NGO responding to HIV/AIDS. Any NGO responding to HIV/AIDS may become a signatory if it endorses the principles contained in the Code.

Scope of implementation

The Code is aspirational. It sets out good practice principles, rather than minimum standards, which we can work towards implementing over time. Signatory NGOs have endorsed all the principles in the Code. However, not all the programming principles in Chapter 4 are applicable to all Supporting NGOs. For example, some will be relevant to development NGOs and others to NGOs working in HIV prevention or treatment, care and support. Signatory NGOs will work to implement the programming principles in the Code relevant to their own work (see sections 5.1 'Signing on' to the Code and 5.2 Implementation of the Code).

Notes

1   *2004 Report on the Global AIDS Epidemic*, Joint United Nations Programme on HIV/AIDS (UNAIDS), p.13. www.unaids.org

2   ibid., *Executive summary – Global Overview.*

3   ibid., p.13.

4   UN Millennium Declaration, Resolution adopted by the General Assembly, 55th Session, 8 September 2000, A/RES/55/2. An overview of the Millennium Development Goals is available at www.un.org

5   Ninety-five per cent of people with HIV/AIDS live in developing countries. *A Commitment to Action for Expanding Access to HIV/AIDS Treatment*, International HIV Treatment Access Coalition, December 2002. Globally, fewer than one in five people at risk of infection has access to basic prevention services. *Access to HIV Prevention: Closing the Gap*, Global Prevention Working Group, May 2003, p.2. www.kff.org

6   Declaration of Commitment on HIV/AIDS, United Nations General Assembly Special Session on HIV/AIDS (UNGASS), 25-27 June 2001. www.un.org

7   *Report of the Secretary General on Progress Towards Implementation of the Declaration of Commitment on HIV/AIDS*, United National General Assembly, August 2002, A/57/227.

8   *Stories from the Front Lines: Experiences and Lessons Learned in the First Two Years of Advocacy around the Declaration of Commitment,* International Council of AIDS Service Organisations (ICASO), September 2003.

9   Steinbrook, R., *After Bangkok – Expanding the Global Response to AIDS*, New England Journal of Medicine, 351;8, p.738. www.nejm.org

10 *2004 Report on the Global AIDS Epidemic*, UNAIDS, p.132.

11 ibid., p.101.

12 *Treating 3 million by 2005 – Making it Happen*, WHO, December 2003. www.who.int

13 The UNAIDS framework known as the 'Three Ones' aims to achieve this. The Three Ones provide that national responses have one agreed HIV/AIDS action framework, one national AIDS coordinating authority with a broad multi-sectoral mandate, and one agreed country-level monitoring and evaluation system.

Guiding Principles

2.1 Introduction

This chapter sets out the guiding principles – human rights, public health and development – that provide the overarching framework for the Code. These principles are then applied in specific terms both to how we do our work (Chapter 3 – Organisational Principles) and to what we do (Chapter 4 – Programming Principles). The guiding principles and organisational principles are relevant to all NGO signatories to the Code. The programming principles are more specific and therefore may apply to different NGOs depending on the nature of their work.

2.2 Core values

The motivation for, and commitment to, responding to HIV/AIDS is underscored by core values that guide both what we do and how we work.

At the centre of our work is our commitment to:

- valuing human life
- respecting the dignity of all people
- respecting diversity and promoting the equality of all people without distinction of any kind, such as sex, race, colour, age, language, religion, political or other opinion, national or social origin, property, birth, physical or mental disability, health status (including HIV/AIDS), sexual orientation or civil, political, social or other status
- preventing and eliminating human suffering
- supporting community values that encourage respect for others and a willingness to work together to find solutions, in the spirit of compassion and mutual support, and
- addressing social and economic inequities and fostering social justice.

These values are common to our work as NGOs in responding to HIV/AIDS, whether we are HIV/AIDS, health, development, human rights or humanitarian NGOs.[1] Many of these same values also find expression in the Universal Declaration of Human Rights.[2]

2.3 Involvement of PLHA and affected communities

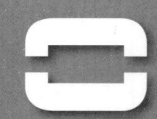 We advocate for the meaningful involvement of PLHA and affected communities in all aspects of the HIV/AIDS response.

At the Paris AIDS Summit in 1994, the principle of greater involvement of people living with or affected by HIV/AIDS (GIPA) was a cornerstone of the Summit's Declaration.[3] GIPA is a specific expression of the right to active, free and meaningful participation.[4] In emphasising GIPA and the right to participation, we recognise that the meaningful involvement of PLHA and affected communities makes a powerful contribution by enabling individuals and communities to draw on their lived experiences in responding to HIV/AIDS. In turn, this contributes to reducing stigma and discrimination and to increasing the effectiveness and appropriateness of the HIV/AIDS response and of our own programmes[5] (see section 3.2 Involvement of PLHA and affected communities).

It is important to acknowledge that many people living with and affected by HIV/AIDS are actively involved in responding to the pandemic – not only within NGOs, but also as policy-makers, activists, healthcare workers, educators, scientists, community leaders and public servants, to name just a few. Nonetheless, there remains a long way to go in fully realising GIPA worldwide. We have a significant role to play in advocating with governments, donors and private and public sector agencies for the meaningful involvement of PLHA and affected communities, as well as in achieving GIPA within our own organisations.

A pyramid of involvement by PLHA

This pyramid models the increasing levels of involvement advocated by GIPA, with the highest level representing complete application of the GIPA principle. Ideally GIPA is applied at all levels of organisation.

Level of involvement

Decision-makers: PLHA participate in decision-making or policy-making bodies, and their inputs are valued equally with all the other members of these bodies.

Experts: PLHA are recognised as important sources of information, knowledge and skills and participate – on the same level as professionals – in the design, adaptation and evaluation of interventions.

Implementers: PLHA carry out real and instrumental roles in interventions, e.g. as carers, peer educators or outreach workers. However, PLHA do not design the intervention or have little say how it is run.

Speakers: PLHA are used as spokespersons in campaigns to change behaviours, or are brought into conferences or meetings to 'share their views' but otherwise do not participate. (This is often perceived as 'token' participation, where the organisers are conscious of the need to be seen as involving PLHA, but do not given them any real power or responsibility.)

Contributors: activities involve PLHA only marginally, generally when the individual affected by HIV/AIDS is already well-known. For example, using an HIV–positive pop star on a poster, or having relatives of someone who has recently died of AIDS speak about that person at public occasions.

Target audiences: activities are aimed at or conducted for PLHA or address them en masse, rather than as individuals.
However, PLHA should be recognised as more than
a) anonymous images on leaflets and posters, or in information, education and communication (IEC) campaigns,
b) people who only receive services, or
c) as 'patients' at this level. They can provide important feedback, which in turn can influence or inform the sources of the information.

Adapted from *From Principles to Practice: Greater Involvement of People Living with or Affected by HIV/AIDS, UNAIDS*, 1999.

2.4 A human rights approach to HIV/AIDS

The AIDS pandemic is destroying the lives and livelihoods of millions of people around the world. The situation is worst in regions and countries where poverty is extensive, gender inequity is pervasive and public services are weak.[6]

In recent years, the devastation caused by HIV/AIDS in many developing countries has brought into stark relief the need to strengthen the link between furthering development goals and addressing the causes of vulnerability to HIV/AIDS and its impacts. HIV/AIDS-specific approaches alone, such as targeted HIV prevention programmes, do not address the underlying causes of vulnerability. Addressing the inequities that drive the epidemic must be an integral part of an effective response.

Poverty both causes vulnerability to HIV infection and increases the severity of the impacts of HIV/AIDS on individuals, households and communities.[7] Gender inequities often affect the capacity of women and girls to negotiate safer sex and compound the impact of the epidemic on them. Many of the impediments to an effective response to HIV/AIDS are linked to the denial of human rights: the rights to equality, information, privacy, health, education and an adequate standard of living. Failure to protect the human rights of PLHA and affected communities has devastating consequences and undermines prevention efforts and access to treatment, care and support. Discrimination against PLHA and affected communities often affects access to employment, housing, health and other services, in turn deepening the personal and social impacts of the epidemic.

The Declaration of Commitment on HIV/AIDS recognises that the realisation of human rights is essential to reducing vulnerability to HIV/AIDS and sets time-bound targets for realising these rights.[8] Experience has shown that public health strategies and human rights protection are mutually reinforcing.[9] A human rights approach provides a common framework for translating international human rights obligations into practical programming, at international and national level, strengthening the effectiveness of both HIV/AIDS-specific programmes and broader health, development and humanitarian responses.[10]

Human rights laws protect individuals and groups from actions that interfere with fundamental freedoms and human dignity.[11] Protecting and promoting human rights has obvious merit intrinsically; however, there is also an increasing recognition that public health often provides an added and compelling justification for safeguarding human rights.[12]

Human rights encompass civil, political, cultural, economic and social rights. It is clear that these rights are interrelated and interdependent. The right to health, for example, cannot be viewed in isolation from the rights to education, housing and employment.

Every country in the world is now party to at least one human rights treaty that addresses health-related rights, including the right to health and a number of rights related to conditions necessary for health.[13] International human rights instruments impose obligations on governments ratifying them to respect, protect and fulfil the rights they set out. While the principle of progressive realisation of human rights acknowledges that the capacity of developing countries to ensure the full realisation of these rights is often constrained by limitations on resources, it also requires governments to take deliberate, concrete and targeted action towards that goal.[14]

Human rights obligations can be used by NGOs to advocate for concrete action by governments. The *HIV/AIDS and Human Rights: International Guidelines*[15] provide detailed and specific guidance on how human rights should be promoted and protected in the context of the specific challenges posed by HIV/AIDS.

We must also be guided by a human rights approach in:
- the way we do our work
- the design, development and implementation of programmes responding to HIV/AIDS, and
- advocating for an environment, including reform of laws and public policy, that protects and promotes the rights of PLHA and affected communities and supports effective programmes (an 'enabling environment'; see section 3.8 Advocacy).

The human rights principles and public health principles outlined below are embodied in the good practice principles outlined in chapters 3 and 4. The human rights principles outlined below identify the principles of particular relevance in responding to HIV/AIDS.

Human rights

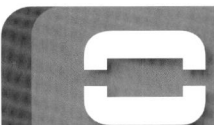 We protect and promote human rights in our work.

The right to health

All people have the right to the enjoyment of the highest attainable standard of physical and mental health. The International Covenant on Economic, Social and Cultural Rights 1966 (ICESCR) provides that states party to the Covenant take steps to achieve the full realisation of this right, including prevention, treatment and control of epidemic, endemic, occupational and other diseases.[16]

The Committee on Economic, Social and Cultural Rights, which monitors the ICESCR convention, has interpreted the 'right to health' to include not only timely and appropriate access to health care, but also as addressing the underlying determinants of health, such as access to safe water, food, nutrition, housing and health-related education and information, including on sexual and reproductive health.[17] In 2003 and 2004, the Commission on Human Rights passed resolutions recognising that access to HIV treatment is fundamental to progressively achieving the right to health and called on governments and international bodies to take specific steps to enable such access.[18]

The right to equality and non-discrimination

The cornerstone of the Universal Declaration of Human Rights 1948 (UDHR) is that 'All human beings are born free and equal in rights and dignity'. This statement of equality of all human beings is closely linked to the right of all people to equal protection of the law and from discrimination.[19] For example, ICESCR prohibits discrimination in access to health care and underlying determinants of health, as well as to means and entitlements for their procurement, on the grounds of race, colour, sex, language, religion, political or other opinion, national or social origin, property, birth, physical or mental disability, health status (including HIV/AIDS), sexual orientation and civil, political, social or other status, which has the intention or effect of adversely affecting the equal enjoyment or exercise of the right to health.[20]

In addition to the above, there are a range of other human rights principles that are relevant in responding to HIV/AIDS.

The right to privacy

No-one shall be subject to arbitrary or unlawful interference with his/her privacy.[21]

The right to information

Everyone has the right to freedom of expression; this right includes freedom to seek, receive and impart information and ideas of all kinds.[22]

The right of participation

Everyone has the right to active, free and meaningful participation.[23]

The right to enjoy the benefits of scientific progress

Everyone has the right to enjoy the benefits of scientific progress and its applications.[24]

Freedom from torture

No-one shall be subject to torture or to cruel, inhuman or degrading treatment or punishment. In particular, no-one shall be subjected to medical or scientific experimentation without free consent.[25]

Freedom of association

Everyone shall have the right to freedom of association with others, including the right to form and join trade unions.[26]

The right to work

Everyone has the right to work, to free choice of employment, to just and favourable conditions of work and to protection against unemployment.[27]

The right to education

Everyone has the right to education, directed to the full development of the human personality and the sense of its dignity, enabling all persons to participate effectively in a free society and promoting understanding, tolerance and friendship among all nations and all racial, ethnic or religious groups.[28]

The right to an adequate standard of living

Everyone has the right to an adequate standard of living, including adequate food, clothing, housing, medical care and necessary social services.[29]

The right to development

Everyone is entitled to participate in, contribute to, and enjoy economic, social, cultural and political development, in which all human rights and fundamental freedoms can be fully realised.[30]

Public health

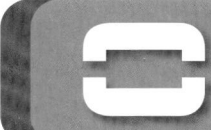 We apply public health principles in our work.

Broad definition of health

The goal of public health is to promote the health of communities. A broad definition of 'health' is required to take into account the social determinants of health, which so significantly affect the achievement of this goal. WHO defines health as a state of complete physical, mental and social well-being, and not merely the absence of disease or infirmity.[31]

Addressing population vulnerability

In order to promote the health of communities at a population level, it is critical to understand the array of factors that place particular populations at risk of HIV transmission or exacerbate the impact of HIV/AIDS, including the social factors that underscore such vulnerability. Understanding the causes of vulnerability and developing service and programme responses that address the needs of specific communities is essential in an effective response to HIV/AIDS.

Evidence-informed approaches

A comprehensive and participatory assessment of populations' needs, in order to identify, understand and address population vulnerability, requires an approach that is informed by evidence. Surveillance, monitoring and risk assessment, encompassing the collection of data related to health status, epidemiological analysis and population health research, provide an essential evidence base for the development and delivery of programmes (see also sections 2.5 Cross-cutting issues: addressing population vulnerability; 3.6 Programme planning, monitoring and evaluation; and 3.9 Research).

Prevention

Public health response to HIV encompasses three levels of prevention activities:
- primary prevention measures to prevent HIV transmission
- secondary prevention measures to ensure early detection and successful management and treatment for PLHA
- tertiary prevention measures to limit the further negative effects of HIV and increase the quality of life of PLHA.

The public health model of primary, secondary and tertiary prevention may not be the language that all NGOs use. Nonetheless, this approach reflects what we do. We work to prevent HIV transmission, provide treatment, care and support, and address the underlying causes of HIV/AIDS and its impacts.

Community organisation

Communities are a vital part of the HIV/AIDS response. Communities must be mobilised, informed and empowered to enable them to increase control over, and to improve, their health. This means that communities must be involved in setting priorities, making decisions, and planning and implementing strategies to achieve better health. At the heart of this process is the empowerment of communities, and their ownership and control of their own endeavours.[32]

Public policy

Public health policy seeks to influence the social conditions that affect health by promoting the use of a scientific knowledge base and an understanding of the determinants of health in the development of public policy, legislation and health systems to provide an enabling environment for effective responses to HIV/AIDS.

Development

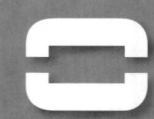

We address the causes of vulnerability to HIV infection and the impacts of HIV/AIDS.

HIV/AIDS has devastating and far-reaching implications for individuals, families, communities and societies. Epidemic diseases are not new, but what sets HIV/AIDS apart is its unprecedented negative impact on the social and economic development of nations most affected by it. In high-prevalence countries, skilled personnel in public, social, education and health care services are becoming ill and dying, undermining the capacity of services to meet demands that continue to escalate as a consequence of HIV/AIDS. The pandemic is reducing labour forces and agricultural productivity, thus exacerbating global poverty and vulnerability to HIV/AIDS infection. Millions of children in developing countries are without adequate care and support, which places additional pressures on families and communities to care for orphans and children made vulnerable by HIV/AIDS (OVC). As parents and care-givers become ill or die, children are increasingly shouldering the burden of generating an income, producing food and taking care of family members who are ill.[33] Women and girls bear a large proportion of the burden of AIDS care, both in the formal care sector and informally in communities. This often leads to girls having to leave school, women having diminished opportunities for economic independence, and women living with HIV/AIDS struggling to meet their own as well as their families' care needs, all of which further entrenches gender inequities.[34]

A human rights approach to HIV/AIDS encompasses the right to development, where all people are entitled to participate in, contribute to, and enjoy economic, social, cultural and political development. It also supports efforts to address the underlying causes of vulnerability to HIV/AIDS and its impacts. The Declaration of Commitment on HIV/AIDS provides explicit commitments to invest in sustainable development in order to alleviate the social and economic impacts of HIV/AIDS, and calls for multi-sectoral strategies, including:

- developing and accelerating the implementation of national poverty eradication strategies to address the impact of HIV/AIDS on household income, livelihoods and access to basic social services, with special focus on individuals, families and communities severely affected by the epidemic;
- reviewing the social and economic impact of HIV/AIDS at all levels of society, especially on women and older people, and particularly on their role as care-givers in families affected by HIV/AIDS, to address their special needs; and
- adjusting and adapting economic and social development policies, including social protection policies, to address the impact of HIV/AIDS on economic growth, the provision of essential economic services, labour productivity, government revenues and deficit-creating pressures on public resources[35] (see also section 4.3 Mainstreaming HIV/AIDS).

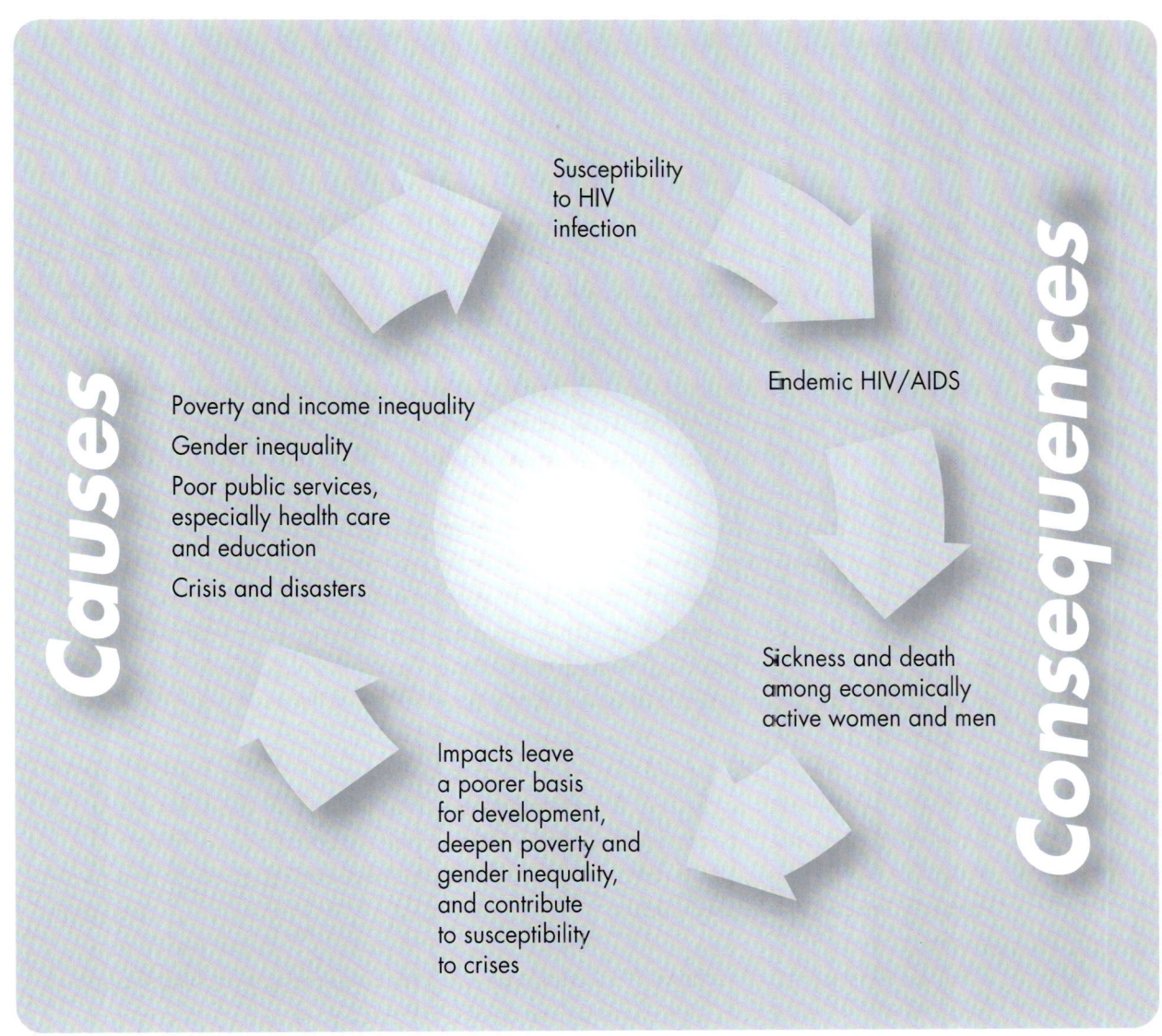

From *Mainstreaming HIV/AIDS in Development and Humanitarian Programmes,* Sue Holden, Oxfam Publishing, 2004.

2.5 Cross-cutting issues: addressing population vulnerability

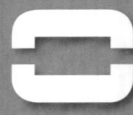

Our programmes are informed by evidence in order to respond to the needs of those most vulnerable to HIV/AIDS and its consequences.

Given the significant differences between HIV/AIDS epidemics around the world, population priorities will vary depending on the nature of the epidemic, including whether there is high, medium or low HIV prevalence and whether the epidemic is widespread or concentrated within specific populations, such as people who inject drugs or men who have sex with men.

One of the key aims of this Code is to articulate the principles, practices and evidence base that underscore successful NGO work in responding to HIV/AIDS and that have global applications. It is not within the scope of the Code to provide detailed programming responses for the diversity of epidemics worldwide. Nonetheless, this section aims to highlight some of the key population groups that need to be considered in our work, depending on the context.

Priority must be given, and resources allocated, to meet the needs of those most vulnerable to HIV/AIDS and its impacts. While PLHA, their families and carers are a consistent priority, populations particularly vulnerable to HIV/AIDS and its impacts will vary from country to country, depending on the nature of the epidemic. This demands that our responses to HIV/AIDS be based on context-specific evidence. We need to understand the epidemiology, the social patterns of sexual activity and injecting drug use and the nature of the impact of HIV/AIDS in any given context.

Attention needs to be paid to the gender dimensions of HIV/AIDS. HIV/AIDS is not only driven by gender inequity – it entrenches it.[36] Women and girls are becoming increasing vulnerable to HIV infection and bear the overwhelming burden of AIDS care, both informally in their families and communities and in the formal care sector.[37] The 'feminisation' of epidemics is starkest where heterosexual sex is the dominant mode of transmission. Women also figure significantly in many countries with epidemics that are concentrated in key populations such as injecting drug users, mobile populations and prisoners.[38]

The population groups considered in this section are clearly not mutually exclusive. This requires that we understand and take account of the multiple factors, such as gender, age, sexuality, ethnicity and socio-economic status, that shape people's lives in ways that influence their vulnerability to HIV/AIDS. Section 5.3 Key resources provides tools that can support the application of these programming principles when working with specific populations.

People living with HIV/AIDS

The impact of HIV/AIDS is felt most strongly, and understood most profoundly, by those living with the disease. The meaningful involvement of PLHA and affected communities makes a powerful contribution to the HIV/AIDS response by empowering people living with HIV/AIDS to draw on their lived experiences. In turn this contributes to reducing stigma and discrimination and increasing the effectiveness and appropriateness of programmes (see section 3.2).

Women and girls and men and boys

Programmes need to recognise and respond to the variety of ways in which gender inequities expose women and girls to the risk of HIV infection, undermine women's access to information, services and programmes, and entrench the subordination of women. In many cultures, unequal power in sexual relationships undermines the capacity of women and girls to exercise control over their sexual choices. One of the most serious manifestations of this inequity is gender-based violence, which can expose women to HIV infection, and fear of which can prevent them from protecting themselves against infection. Legislation often restricts the right of women to own or inherit property, entrenching their economic dependence on men, and limiting their capacity to refuse sex or negotiate condom use. A gendered approach to HIV/AIDS requires advocating for a legislative and policy environment that promotes the rights of women and girls, in order to shift the dynamics that underscore women's subordinate position in society and sexual relationships (see good practice principles in advocating for an enabling environment in sections 4.2 HIV/AIDS programming on page 63 and 4.3 Mainstreaming HIV/AIDS on page 83).

To reduce the spread and minimise the impact of HIV/AIDS, inequities between men and women must be reduced. This must necessarily involve men and boys as well as women and girls. Given the power men often have in society, communities, families and sexual relationships, there is a growing recognition of the need for programmes for men and boys that challenge gender roles and norms, enabling them to change their attitudes and behaviours that affect the vulnerability of women and girls. There is also a need to address the ways in which gender roles and norms undermine men's ability to access health programmes, including sexual health, HIV prevention and treatment, care and support.[39]

Children and young people

Young people continue to make up a significant proportion of new infections each year, with 38 per cent of PLHA worldwide now under the age of 25.[40] We need to recognise and meet the needs of the growing population of young people living with HIV/AIDS. Sub-populations of young people are particularly vulnerable to infection, including young women, young men who have sex with men, young people who inject drugs, and sexually exploited children.[41] Many young people do not know how to protect themselves from HIV, and there are significant social and cultural barriers that impede the widespread availability of appropriate sexual health and HIV education for young people.[42]

There is also a clear cycle of vulnerability in relation to orphans and children affected by HIV/AIDS. An estimated 14 million children worldwide have lost one or both parents to AIDS.[43] A holistic response, including care in the community, is needed to address their needs, and this in turn can reduce their vulnerability to HIV infection.[44]

Older people

Older people are both infected and affected by HIV/AIDS, but far too often their specific needs are overlooked. Data on infection rates among people over 50 are inadequate, yet the data that are available indicate rising infection rates among older people. With the expanding availability of ARVs, more people will be living with HIV/AIDS and their needs are likely to change as they grow older. In high-prevalence countries in particular, older people are often the primary carers for their adult children who have HIV/AIDS and/or children orphaned or made vulnerable by their parents' ill health or untimely death. Age-, gender- and HIV/AIDS-related stigma plays a role in older men and women being overlooked in programming.[45]

Men who have sex with men (MSM), including gay men

Sex between men has been the predominant mode of transmission in some countries. However, it is also a factor in all HIV epidemics, though it is often statistically hidden and officially denied.[46] In recent decades there have been significant advances in decriminalising sex between men in many countries. Nonetheless, laws that criminalise or otherwise stigmatise or discriminate against MSM are contrary to human rights law and continue to drive the spread of HIV by alienating such men from access to prevention, treatment, care and support programmes.[47] Programmes need to be appropriate for MSM and enable them to protect themselves from HIV infection and respond to discrimination. Advocacy efforts need to be directed to law reform and addressing the social stigmatisation that increases the vulnerability of MSM.

Generally, the term 'men who have sex with men (MSM)' is used throughout the Code to include gay men. However, it is important to note that the needs and experiences of gay men and men who have sex with men but who may not identify as gay are different, and require responses that are appropriate to those differing needs and experiences.

Sex workers and their clients

The stigma associated with sex work in many countries around the world creates significant barriers to sexual health and HIV prevention efforts among sex workers and their clients. While sex work has been decriminalised in some countries, it remains illegal in many more. Even where knowledge about safe sex practices is high among sex workers, the prevailing power dynamics, entrenched by gender, legal and social inequities, make it difficult to put that knowledge into practice. With this in mind, programmes, services and advocacy efforts need to be appropriate for sex workers and their clients. Strategies are required to promote an environment which supports access to treatment for HIV and other sexually transmitted infections (STIs). Supporting sex workers, including through collective action, empowers them to negotiate transactions, and address the health and social contexts that increase their vulnerability to HIV infection.

People who inject drugs

HIV transmission through injecting drug use accounts for approximately 10 per cent of HIV infections globally and is a dominant factor driving HIV infection rates in many countries.[48]

Injecting drug use is a major factor in epidemics in Asia, North America, Western Europe, parts of Latin America, and in the Middle East and Northern Africa. In some Eastern European countries, especially the countries of the former Soviet Union, injecting drug use is driving an epidemic among young people.[49]

The illegality and stigma associated with injecting drug use invariably lead to discrimination against people who use drugs and create barriers to accessing services.[50] Failure to protect the human rights of people who inject drugs makes them afraid to access health and related support services, leading to negative health outcomes and undermining HIV prevention efforts.[51] A comprehensive range of services and programmes is needed in order to respond effectively to the harms associated with injecting drug use, including education programmes that reduce the risk of HIV infection among those who inject drugs (as well as those that deter people from drug use), access to clean needles and syringes, drug treatment programmes, and appropriate healthcare services. Concerted efforts must be made to ensure support for, and availability of, the full complement of services and programmes that reach and involve people who inject drugs.

Transgender people

Transgender people face stigma and discrimination, which exacerbate their HIV risk. There are few transgender-sensitive HIV/AIDS programmes. Social marginalisation can result in the denial of health, education, employment and housing opportunities. Access to treatment, care and support is often limited due to fear of a person's transgender status being revealed, lack of knowledge about the healthcare needs of transgender people, and discrimination.[52]

Prisoners

Correctional facilities, such as adult gaols and juvenile detention centres, are commonly characterised by concentrated populations of people living with HIV/AIDS, where injecting drug use, tattooing and consensual and forced sex commonly occur, in an environment where there is limited and often no access to the means of preventing the spread of HIV or to education programmes on HIV prevention.[53] This has significant consequences not only for prisoners themselves but also for the families and communities to whom they return, often after relatively short terms of imprisonment. Attempts to reduce drug use by mandatory drug screening have often had counter-productive results.[54] Programmes need to address the specific risks of HIV infection in prisons and meet the often complex health needs of prisoners, including those living with HIV/AIDS.[55]

Mobile populations: internally displaced people, refugees, migrant and mobile workers

The spread of HIV/AIDS across communities, countries and continents is testimony to linkages between population movement and the growing epidemic. There is increasing recognition that the mobility of people, whether displaced by conflict or natural disasters, or to access work, can create particular kinds of vulnerability to HIV/AIDS and its consequences.[56] People move, voluntarily and involuntarily; temporarily, seasonally and permanently.

Mobility increases vulnerability to HIV/AIDS, both for those who are mobile and for their partners back home. Migrant and mobile workers[57] are often more vulnerable to HIV infection because of isolation resulting from stigma and discrimination and differences in language and culture; separation from regular sexual partners; lack of support and friendship; and lack of access to health and social services.[58] Where these factors are combined with lack of legal protection, vulnerability to HIV infection is further increased. Effective responses to the vulnerability of mobile populations must include cross-border and regional responses, involving partners in source, transit and destination countries; culturally and linguistically appropriate outreach programmes; and advocacy efforts to protect and promote the human rights of, and where necessary improve the legal status of, migrant and mobile workers.[59]

At the end of 2001, over 70 different countries were experiencing an emergency situation of some kind, resulting in over 50 million people being affected worldwide.[60] The conditions that arise in emergencies such as armed conflict and natural disasters – social instability, poverty, displacement of populations, gender-based violence – are also the conditions that favour the spread of HIV infection. There is increasing recognition that humanitarian programmes need to both integrate HIV/AIDS-specific responses, such as making condoms available, and adapt interventions to better address the underlying causes of vulnerability to HIV/AIDS and its consequences in emergency settings[61] (see section 3.4 Mainstreaming HIV/AIDS).

Notes

1   See, for example, the outline of humanitarian values of the International Federation of Red Cross and Red Crescent Societies at www.ifrc.org

2   The Universal Declaration of Human Rights (1948). www.unhchr.ch

3   The Declaration of the Paris AIDS Summit (1994) is set out in *From Principle to Practice: Greater Involvement of People Living with or Affected by HIV/AIDS (GIPA)*, UNAIDS Best Practice Collection, September 1999. www.unaids.org, search by title

4   See Section 2.4 regarding the right to participation.

5   Levene, J., *Community Mobilisation and Participatory Approaches: Reviewing Impact and Good Practice for HIV/AIDS Programming*, International HIV/AIDS Alliance, November 2004.

6   Collins, J. and Rau, B., *AIDS in the Context of Development*, United Nations Research Institute for Social Development (UNRISD) Programme on Social Policy and Development, Paper Number 4, Geneva, UNRISD and UNAIDS, 2000, p.6. www.unrisd.org

7   Holden, S., *AIDS on the Agenda: Adapting Development and Humanitarian Programmes to Meet the Challenges of HIV/AIDS*, ActionAid, Oxfam GB and Save the Children UK, 2003. For a detailed discussion of HIV/AIDS as a development issue, see pp.9-38.
    www.oxfam.org.uk

8   Declaration of Commitment on HIV/AIDS, United Nations General Assembly Special Session on HIV/AIDS (UNGASS), 25-27 June 2001.

9   *2004 Report on the Global AIDS Epidemic*, Joint United Nations Programme on HIV/AIDS (UNAIDS), pp.123-127. www.unaids.org. For examples, see section 4.2 of the Code on voluntary counselling and testing and addressing stigma and discrimination.

10 Patterson, D., *Programming HIV/AIDS: A Human Rights Approach. A Tool for International Development and Community Based Organizations Responding to HIV/AIDS*, Canadian HIV/AIDS Legal Network, 2004.
    www.aidslaw.ca

11 *25 Questions and Answers on Health and Human Rights*, World Health Organisation (WHO), Health and Human Rights Publication Series Issue No.1, July 2002, p.9. www.who.int

12 *HIV/AIDS and Human Right: International Guidelines*, Office of the United Nations High Commissioner for Human Rights (OHCHR) and the Joint United Nations Programme on HIV/AIDS (UNAIDS), 1998, www.ohchr.org

13 *25 Questions and Answers on Health and Human Rights*, p.14.

14 International Covenant on Economic, Social and Cultural Rights (ICESCR), Article 2(1); ICESCR General Comment 3 on the nature of state parties' obligations, Fifth Session 1990 (E/1991/23).

15 *HIV/AIDS and Human Right: International Guidelines*, OHCHR and UNAIDS, 1998 and *HIV/AIDS and Human Right: International Guidelines – Revised Guideline 6*, 2002, both at www.ohchr.org

16 ICESCR, article 12. As of November 2003, 148 countries had ratified the ICESCR.

17 In May 2000 the Committee adopted a General Comment on the right to health. General Comments serve to clarify the nature and content of individual rights and the obligations of governments. www.unhchr.ch
Also see *The Protection of Human Rights in the Context of HIV/AIDS*, Commission on Human Rights resolution 2003/47: www.unhchr.ch; and the reports of the UN Special Rapporteur on the Right to Health: www.unhchr.ch

18 See the Commission on Human Rights' resolutions in 2004 on Access to Medication in the Context of Pandemics such as HIV/AIDS, Tuberculosis and Malaria (2004/26) and The Right to Health (2004/27) both at www.unhchr.ch. Also see Access to Medication in the Context of Pandemics such as HIV/AIDS, Tuberculosis and Malaria, Commission on Human Rights resolution 2003/29, April 2003. www.unhchr.ch

19 Universal Declaration of Human Rights (UDHR), articles 1 and 7; International Covenant on Civil and Political Rights 1966 (ICCPR), article 26; ICESCR article 2. The rights of equality and non-discrimination are also reflected in conventions which focus on the rights of women and children. See the Convention on the Elimination of All Forms of Discrimination Against Women 1979 (CEDAW) and the Convention on the Rights of the Child 1989 (CRC) respectively.

20 See The Committee on Economic, Social and Cultural Rights General Comment 14, on the right to health, footnote 17 above.

21 ICCPR, article 17; CEDAW, article 16; CRC article 40.

22 UDHR, article 19; ICCPR, article 19.2; CEDAW, articles 10, 14, 16; CRC, articles 13, 17, 24.

23 ICCPR, article 25; ICESCR, article 15; CEDAW, articles 7, 8, 13, 14; International Convention on the Elimination of All Forms of Racial Discrimination 1963 (CERD), article 5; CRC, articles 3, 9, 12.

24 ICESCR, article 15.

25 ICCPR, article 17; CRC, article 37.

26 ICCPR, article 22; CERD article 5; CRC article 15.

27 UDHR, article 23; ICESCR, articles 6.2, 7(a).

28 ICESCR, article 13; CRC, articles 19, 24, 28, 33; CERD, article 5; CEDAW, articles 10, 16; CROC, articles 19, 24, 28, 33.

29 UDHR, article 25; ICESCR, article 11.

30 Declaration on the Rights to Development (1986), www.unhchr.ch

31 Preamble to the Constitution of the World Health Organisation, as adopted by the International Health Conference, New York, 19-22 June 1946.

32 Ottawa Charter for Health Promotion, 1986. www.who.dk

33 *Children on the Brink 2004: A Joint Report on Orphans Estimates and Program Strategies,* UNAIDS, UNICEF and USAID, July 2002, pp.9-11. www.unicef.org

34 Tallis, V., *Gender and HIV/AIDS: Overview Report*, Bridge Development and Gender, September 2002, p.24.

35 Declaration of Commitment on HIV/AIDS, (UNGASS), 2001, paragraph 68.

36 *Gender and HIV/AIDS: Overview Report*, Bridge Development and Gender, September 2002, p.1. www.ids.ac.uk

37 UNAIDS statistics indicate that in 1997, 41 per cent of PLHA were women, but by 2001 the proportion had increased to 50 per cent. *Gender and HIV/AIDS: Overview Report*, p.12, p.24.

38 *2004 Report on the Global AIDS Epidemic*, UNAIDS, p.22.

39 *Working with Men, Responding to AIDS: Gender, Sexuality, and HIV – A Case Study Collection*, The International HIV/AIDS Alliance, 2003. www.aidsalliance.org

40 *The Tip of the Iceberg: The Global Impact of HIV/AIDS on Youth*, The Henry J Kaiser Foundation, July 2002. www.kff.org

41 For example, new infections among girls are as much as five to six times higher than among boys in some hard-hit countries. *The Tip of the Iceberg: The Global Impact of HIV/AIDS on Youth*, p.7.

42   See *HIV/AIDS and the Rights of the Child*, General Comment No.3, Committee on the Rights of the Child, March 2003. www.unhchr.ch

43   *Report on the Global HIV/AIDS Epidemic 2002*, UNAIDS, p.133.

44   See Section 4.3 Mainstreaming HIV/AIDS.

45   *HIV/AIDS and Ageing: A Briefing Paper*, HelpAge International, May 2003. www.helpage.org

46   Data from countries as diverse as India, Mexico and Thailand confirm that men who have unprotected sex with men also have unprotected sex with women. *Report on the Global HIV/AIDS Epidemic 2002, UNAIDS*, pp.91-92.

47   *HIV/AIDS and Human Right: International Guidelines*, 1998 and *HIV/AIDS and HIV/AIDS and Human Right: International Guidelines – Revised Guideline 6*, 2002, both at www.ohchr.org

48   *Drug use and HIV/AIDS*, UNAIDS, June 2001.

49   *Report on the Global HIV/AIDS Epidemic 2002*, p.94.

50   *HIV and AIDS-Related Stigmatization, Discrimination and Denial: Forms, Contexts and Determinants*, UNAIDS, June 2000. www.unaids.org

51   See, for example, *Lessons Not Learnt: Human Rights Abuses and HIV/AIDS in the Russian Federation*, www.hrw.org and *Not Enough Graves: The War on Drugs, HIV/AIDS, and Violations of Human Rights*, www.hrw.org, Human Rights Watch, 2004.

52   *Transgender and HIV/AIDS* www.surgeongeneral.gov; *National Indigenous Gay and Transgender Project – Consultation Report and Sexual Heath Strategy*, Australian Federation of AIDS Organizations, www.afao.com.au

53   *Report on the Global HIV/AIDS Epidemic 2002*, pp. 97-98.

54   Research into mandatory screening in UK prisons found that inmates shifted from smoking marijuana, which is detectable in urine for several weeks, to injecting heroin, which is undetectable in urine after one to two days. *Report on the Global HIV/AIDS Epidemic 2002*, p.97.

55   Davies, R., Prison's Second Death Row, The Lancet, Vol 364, July 2004, www.aidslaw.ca; and information sheets on HIV/AIDS in prisons, Canadian HIV/AIDS Legal Network, www.aidslaw.ca

56   *Population Mobility and AIDS, UNAIDS Technical Update*, UNAIDS 2001. www.unaids.org

57   Mobile workers include truck drivers, traders, military personnel and seafarers.

58   *Population Mobility and HIV/AIDS*, International Organisation for Migration, July 2004. www.iom.int

59   See also *Focus: AIDS and Mobile Populations, in the Report on the Global HIV/AIDS Epidemic 2002*, UNAIDS, pp.114-119.

60   *Guidelines for HIV/AIDS Interventions in Emergency Settings*, Inter-Agency Standing Committee, 2003. www.humanitarianinfo.org

61   *Guidelines for HIV/AIDS Interventions in Emergency Settings* and The Sphere Project: *Humanitarian Charter and Minimum Standards in Disaster Response*, 2nd Edition, 2004. www.sphereproject.org

Organisational Principles

3.1 Introduction

This chapter provides good practice principles to guide how we do our work. These principles demonstrate, with a greater degree of specificity, our commitment to the guiding principles set out in Chapter 2. They also provide the foundation for effective programming, outlined in Chapter 4. Some of these good practice principles apply specifically to the work of Supporting NGOs, while others are applicable to any NGO that has or may wish to become a signatory to this Code (see section 1.6 Who the Code is for).

3.2 Involvement of PLHA and affected communities

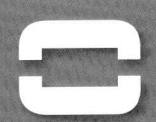 We foster active and meaningful involvement of PLHA and affected communities in our work.

PLHA and affected communities need to be involved in a variety of roles at different levels in NGOs, including as decision-makers on governing boards; as managers, programmers, providers and participants in the design, implementation and evaluation of programmes and services; as decision-makers, advocates and campaigners in policy and advocacy; and as planners, speakers and participants in meetings, conferences and other forums.

In fostering meaningful involvement of PLHA and affected communities within our own organisations and in partnerships with organisations and networks of PLHA and affected communities, we need to:

- create an organisational environment that fosters non-discrimination and values the contribution of PLHA and affected communities
- recognise and foster involvement of the diverse range of PLHA and affected communities (see section 2.5 Cross-cutting issues: addressing population vulnerability)
- ensure involvement in a variety of roles at different levels within our organisations
- define roles and their associated responsibilities; assess what a particular role requires, and the capacity of individuals to fulfil the role; and provide the necessary organisational support, including financial
- ensure organisational policies and practice provide timely access to information to enable participation, preparation and input, before programmatic and policy decisions are made
- ensure workplace policies and practices recognise the health and related needs of PLHA and affected communities and create an enabling environment that supports their involvement (see section 3.5 Organisational mission and management)
- ensure, when seeking PLHA and affected community representatives, that PLHA and affected community organisations and networks have strategies for accountability to their members and processes for ensuring that the views put forward represent their members
- resource and support capacity-building within PLHA and affected community organisations and networks, and
- fund and/or advocate for funding of PLHA and affected community organisations to ensure they have the resources to build capacity and empower others within their own networks.

3.3 Multi-sectoral partnerships

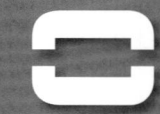

We build and sustain partnerships to support coordinated and comprehensive responses to HIV/AIDS.

No single sector can respond effectively to HIV/AIDS. Multi-sectoral partnerships at all levels, from global to local, are essential in bringing together the necessary expertise, skills, leverage and coordination needed to respond effectively to HIV/AIDS.[1] Governments, public and private sector agencies (such as health, development and scientific communities), donors and a diverse and vibrant civil society, including NGOs and people living with and affected by HIV/AIDS, are essential to a comprehensive and coordinated approach. As we work to scale up our responses, partnerships improve programming by building on the existing infrastructure and expertise of different sectors, enabling integration of HIV/AIDS responses within broader development, health, humanitarian and human rights work, and supporting a comprehensive response in addressing the causes of vulnerability to HIV/AIDS and its consequences.[2] We also need to foster partnerships with governments, policy-makers, the media, and public and private sector agencies, in order to promote an enabling environment for effective responses to HIV/AIDS (see Section 3.8 Advocacy).

We need to foster strategic partnerships that support coordinated and comprehensive programming by:
- establishing mechanisms for assessing and reaching consensus about major unmet need in a given context, including mapping of available programmes and identifying gaps in types of programmes and services or gaps in meeting the needs of particular communities vulnerable to HIV/AIDS
- identifying those organisations or agencies best placed to address unmet need within a given context
- identifying and addressing organisational and competitive obstacles to effective cooperation
- undertaking joint programming or scaling up initiatives in partnership, to enable pooling of resources and expertise and build on existing relationships of trust between different organisations and within communities
- identifying opportunities and acting on or advocating for mainstreaming HIV/AIDS programming within appropriate settings, such as within the education system, poverty reduction initiatives and disaster relief programmes
- ensuring integration of HIV/AIDS with other related health initiatives, such as sexual and reproductive health, malaria and tuberculosis programmes, and
- fostering cross-fertilisation of organisational methods and approaches by sharing lessons learned about successful programming and what has proved effective in scaling up those programmes.

3.4 Governance

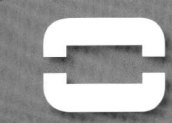 We have transparent governance and are accountable to our communities/constituencies.

Governance bodies need to have clear written policies, which are effectively implemented in practice, and which address the following:
- appointment and termination of members of the governing body
- identification and mitigation of conflicts of interest
- defined roles and responsibilities of the governing body, both individually and jointly, including strategic planning, financial probity and oversight of quality assurance
- guidance on how the strategic responsibilities of the governing body are delegated to operational management
- accountability and reporting arrangements both internally and to donors, NGO partners and communities, where applicable[3]

■ a mandate from communities, whether geographical or population-based, where a supporting NGO provides services and programmes or undertakes advocacy initiatives to a defined community, such as through general elections or the appointment of designated community representatives to the governance body.

3.5 Organisational mission and management

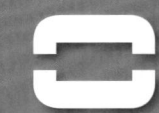 We have a clear mission, supported by strategic objectives that are achieved through good management.

We need to have a clear statement of mission, supported by a statement of values that underpin our work (see section 2.2 Core values). Effective strategic and operational planning, together with effective human resources and financial systems, are essential to support the achievement of our mission. Strategic objectives, over a defined period, need to be informed by an assessment of the HIV/AIDS situation(s) in the country or region concerned, the range of institutional responses that already exist and our own capacity, in order to determine what gaps exist in programming and whether we are best placed to address them (see section 3.3 Multi-sectoral partnerships). Operational planning, which includes clear timeframes and performance indicators, is needed to support the achievement of strategic objectives, as are the allocation of financial and human resources needed to meet these indicators, and a strategic approach to human resources management. Operational plans need to be linked to programme plans and to individual work plans.

Human resources

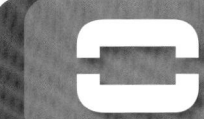 We value, support and effectively manage our human resources.

Our strategic and operational plans need to provide a strategic approach to human resources management, including:
- explicitly valuing staff and volunteer contributions
- allocating sufficient human and financial resources to achieve the objectives set, and
- clear management responsibility for staff and volunteer support, development and well-being.

Our human resources policies and procedures need to be effectively implemented to ensure:
- fair, transparent and effective recruitment and selection of staff and volunteers, including equal opportunity of employment
- consistent and clear guidance to staff regarding roles and responsibilities, including job description and development and regular review of staff work plans
- assessment of human resource capacity, linked to strategic planning
- organisational learning by supporting the training and development of staff and volunteers, and
- security, safety and health of staff and volunteers.

Our human resources policies and practices need to create an enabling organisational environment for responding to HIV/AIDS by:
- developing and implementing policies and procedures that promote inclusion of and commitment to the employment of PLHA and affected communities, such as affirmative action strategies that address underlying obstacles to meaningful participation and acknowledge the value of the involvement of PLHA and affected communities in a wide range of roles
- promoting a non-discriminatory workplace through awareness raising and training on stigma and discrimination, together with grievance procedures to respond to discrimination
- providing terms and conditions of employment that cover bereavement leave and leave for carers, long-term illness provision, reasonable accommodation of staff health needs (such as flexible work practices) and confidentiality
- developing and implementing policies and procedures for universal infection control, including provision of equipment and staff training
- advocating for health insurance products covering HIV/AIDS-related conditions,[4]
- providing access to voluntary testing and counselling (VCT) and prevention, treatment, care and support services and programmes,[5] and
- reducing vulnerability of the organisation to the impact of HIV/AIDS, for example through long-term workforce planning.[6]

Organisational capacity

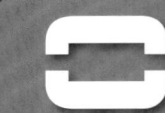

We develop and maintain the organisational capacity necessary to support effective responses to HIV/AIDS.

We need to enable our staff and volunteers to develop and maintain the necessary capacity to effectively carry out their work, including:

- understanding the nature of stigma and discrimination, and the rights of PLHA and affected communities
- examining their own attitudes and beliefs and the impact these may have on their ability to provide non-judgemental, inclusive processes and programmes
- understanding and applying the organisational policies that ensure the rights of PLHA and affected communities and promote participation in programmes
- understanding the diversity of needs within the communities they work with and implementing effective programming to prevent HIV transmission; meet the treatment, care and support needs of PLHA and affected communities; and address the causes and consequences of vulnerability to HIV/AIDS
- empowering individuals and communities to understand their own risks and needs, make informed decisions and develop the necessary skills to protect themselves and others from HIV infection and/or to meet their own treatment, care and support needs
- empowering individuals and communities to take action in response to stigma and discrimination and/or to make appropriate referrals
- designing, delivering and evaluating programmes in their particular fields of expertise, and
- continually improving programming and work practices through effective programme planning, monitoring and evaluation cycles.

Financial resources

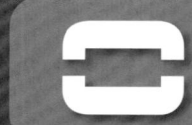

We manage financial resources in an efficient, transparent and accountable manner.

We need to manage financial resources in an efficient, transparent and accountable manner by ensuring:

- that fund-raising strategies and funding sources are consistent with and supportive of our mission
- there is systemic preparation of budgets linked to strategic, operational and programme plans
- that budgeting supports the human resources and organisational capacity necessary to achieve our mission[7]
- there are internal control systems that enable production of regular, consistent and reliable financial information, which complies with legal requirements

- there are internal accounting systems that provide regular financial reports, in a consistent and accessible format
- that financial reports can be utilised to track resources, monitor programme spending against budget allocation and assess the cost-effectiveness of programmes
- there is an efficient grant programming system and provision of finance and administrative technical support, where funding is provided to partner NGOs
- there is regular financial reporting to management, the governing board, donors and communities/constituencies, and annual financial auditing of accounts, and
- there is transparent annual reporting, including statutory reports where required.[8]

3.6 Programme planning, monitoring and evaluation

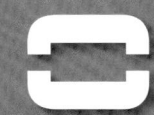 **We select appropriate partners in a transparent manner.**

Transparent selection systems are needed to ensure identification of partner NGOs that:
- are the most appropriate to achieve the programme objectives
- have the necessary financial and programmatic capacity to manage activities, or can be supported to develop financial and programmatic capacity, and
- are appropriate to work with identified beneficiary communities, including assessment of community credibility.

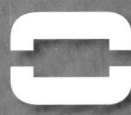

We plan, monitor and evaluate programmes for effectiveness and in response to community need.

Efforts to better understand and improve the effectiveness of HIV prevention, treatment, care and support services and programmes have produced an impressive body of knowledge and resources to inform planning, monitoring and evaluation.[9] Programme plans need to set clear objectives, timeframes, performance indicators and reporting requirements, and allocate the financial and human resources needed to meet programme objectives.

Programme objectives and priorities need to be informed by evidence drawing on:
- relevant epidemiological, social and behavioural research data
- relevant programme evaluation findings, and
- assessment of community need, including mapping of available services and programmes to determine gaps in programmes and services or gaps in meeting the needs of particular communities vulnerable to HIV/AIDS.

Programme plans need to incorporate monitoring and evaluation into the programming planning cycle by:
- setting programme objectives at the outset that are appropriate for monitoring and evaluation of the programme
- developing monitoring indicators and using them to guide systematic collection of information, including qualitative data over time, to assess whether the programme is proceeding according to plan, and whether there are obstacles that need to be addressed
- gathering relevant baseline data as a basis for assessing the progress and impact of programming
- evaluating programmes to assess their quality, efficiency and effectiveness
- regularly utilising data gathered and adjusting programmes over time to ensure flexibility and responsiveness of programming, and
- utilising programme evaluation findings to inform future programmes.

The programme plans of Supporting NGOs need to include technical support for partner NGOs on:
- HIV/AIDS-related issues as required by specific programmes
- programming design, implementation, monitoring and evaluation, and
- organisational development, including strategic planning, financial and administrative systems, and human resource strategies to promote effective management of staff and organisational learning.

3.7 Access and equity

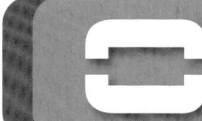 Our programmes are non-discriminatory, accessible and equitable.

The term 'discrimination' is used when people are treated adversely, either by treating them the same when their needs are different, or by treating them differently when they should be treated the same.[10] Equity in programming requires that resources are allocated and programmes are developed in response to the needs of both individuals and communities.

Accessibility of services alone is insufficient to respond to the diverse needs of PLHA and affected communities. Programmes that are generic in nature, assuming that communities are reached by the same approach or type of service, often reflect and entrench social inequities. To ensure access and equity, programmes need to be tailored to meet the particular needs of PLHA and affected communities, depending on the context (see section 2.5 Cross-cutting issues: addressing population vulnerability). For example, HIV prevention programmes, for men and women, need to address gender stereotypes, norms, attitudes and practices in order to address underlying gender inequities that increase the vulnerability of women and girls to HIV infection. So too, gender inequities that impede access to services and programmes for women, including those living with HIV/AIDS, need to be understood and addressed.

Programmes need to be respectful of the culture of individuals, minorities, peoples and communities, and sensitive to gender and life-cycle requirements. Equity of and access to services and programmes are best achieved by actively involving PLHA and affected communities not only in the design and delivery of programmes, but also in a wide variety of roles within NGOs (see sections 2.3 and 3.2 Involvement of PLHA and affected communities).

Access to programmes and services needs to be supported by workplace polices and practices that ensure that:
- the rights of PLHA and affected communities are respected[11]
- the rights of service users are clearly articulated and promoted to communities, particularly those most marginalised
- people have access to appropriate information to enable them to understand the implications of participation, and freely decide whether or not they wish to participate[12]
- the rights of service users are supported by understandable and accessible complaints mechanisms
- confidentiality is protected, thereby promoting an environment where PLHA and affected communities feel able to access information and programmes and actively participate in the HIV/AIDS response[13] and
- PLHA and affected communities are actively involved in a wide range of roles within the organisation.

3.8 Advocacy

Advocacy is a method and a process of influencing decision-makers and public perceptions about an issue of concern, and mobilising community action to achieve social change, including legislative and policy reform, to address the concern.

The term **enabling environment** is used to refer to an environment where laws and public policy protect and promote the rights of PLHA and affected communities, support effective programmes, reduce vulnerability to HIV/AIDS and address its consequences.

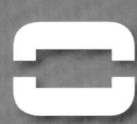

We advocate for an enabling environment that protects and promotes the rights of PLHA and affected communities and supports effective programming.

Laws, policies, social norms and community attitudes and perceptions shape the environment in which we respond to HIV/AIDS. Our efforts to address both the causes and consequences of the HIV/AIDS pandemic require fundamental social change (see section 2.4 A human rights approach to HIV/AIDS). Advocacy efforts may be focused at local, national and international level, with the aim of creating and sustaining an environment where laws and public policy protect and promote the rights of PLHA and affected communities, support effective programmes and reduce vulnerability to HIV/AIDS and its consequences. The Declaration of Commitment on HIV/AIDS, international human rights instruments and the *HIV/AIDS and Human Rights: International Guidelines* provide a blueprint for reform and invaluable tools for advocating national action.[14]

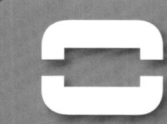

We plan, monitor and evaluate advocacy efforts for effectiveness and in response to community need.

While there is a wealth of resources devoted to monitoring and evaluating the impact of different types of programme interventions, there is comparatively little in the way of monitoring and evaluating advocacy activities. The causality between advocacy efforts and changes in law and policy and in social norms is often difficult to measure. We have much to contribute to improving knowledge in this area.

In planning, implementing, monitoring and evaluating advocacy activities, we need to:
- actively involve PLHA, affected communities and community and opinion leaders[15]
- map the environment to determine the factors that may affect advocacy processes and outcomes, such as leadership, HIV/AIDS policy environment and legislative impediments to effective advocacy or HIV/AIDS programmes[16]
- draw on experiences in the provision of programmes and services to inform advocacy priorities
- set clear objectives about what legal, policy or social change is being sought
- identify and develop strategic partnerships with organisations, institutions and networks that share common goals and can lend support to achieving objectives by increasing our influence and capacity to achieve change through joint action[17]
- determine the most appropriate advocacy methods for achieving objectives, such as media campaigns and lobbying policy-makers
- identify and build relationships with the target audiences needed to achieve objectives, such as political leaders, religious and community leaders, policy-makers and the media
- use experiences drawn from programmes and services to support the rationale for changes sought[18]
- develop evaluation methods that define information to be collected and a method of analysis to determine whether objectives are achieved
- collect qualitative data to track the external environment to assess the effectiveness of advocacy efforts, including media reports, policy statements of target audience, meetings and discussions
- collect qualitative data on the process of undertaking advocacy efforts, such as effectiveness of partnerships and alliances, 'packaging' messages and the use of evidence
- collect quantitative data from target audiences, programme implementers, strategic partners and beneficiaries of advocacy efforts about both the processes used and the impact of advocacy activities
- use the data gathered to assess the extent to which advocacy efforts have affected awareness about the issues; influenced the organisation's credibility as an advocate; made a contribution to debate; changed laws and policy; influenced the attitudes or beliefs of opinion leaders; and affected the lives of PLHA and affected communities
- use the information gathered to assess the effectiveness of processes used, including effectiveness of partnerships, involvement of PLHA and affected communities and organisational advocacy capacity,[19] and
- use the evaluation of advocacy work to inform future advocacy planning and share lessons learned with partners.

3.9 Research

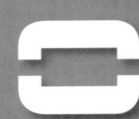

We undertake and/or advocate for adequate and appropriate research to ensure responses to HIV/AIDS are informed by evidence.

The results of good-quality, appropriate and up-to-date research data must guide our actions to enable an effective response to HIV/AIDS (see Public health in section 2.4). Research must include:

- epidemiological, social and behavioural research
- operational research (programme evaluation) to inform programming and policy development[20]
- basic and clinical research into new and/or improved therapeutic, diagnostic and preventive products and technologies (e.g. safety and efficacy of HIV/AIDS-related treatments, fixed-dose combinations of ARVs, cheap and easy-to-use diagnostic tests, microbicides and preventive vaccines),[21] and
- research related to the clinical management of HIV/AIDS, including co-infection with other diseases, to advance best practice in health management.

We need to undertake and/or advocate for adequate and appropriate research to ensure that responses to HIV/AIDS are informed by evidence, by:

- advocating for the involvement of PLHA and affected communities in setting research priorities, in designing and conducting research and analysing the results of research
- advocating for ethical research and/or participation in ethical review processes in order to protect and promote the human rights of people participating in research[22]
- identifying situations where available epidemiological data is inadequate
- advocating for improvements in the type of data collected and/or the systems for collection and reporting to provide an accurate picture of risk and impacts in a given population
- identifying where social and behavioural research is needed in order to better understand the risks associated with HIV infection, the needs of PLHA and affected communities, and the social, political, cultural and economic factors that influence HIV transmission, treatment, care and other aspects of HIV/AIDS in a given context[23]
- undertaking and/or advocating for research to improve the appropriateness and effectiveness of programme interventions, such as evaluation of the impact of efforts to scale up programmes (see also sections 3.6 Programme planning, monitoring and evaluation, 3.10 Scaling up and 4.3 Mainstreaming HIV/AIDS)
- undertaking and/or advocating for research to improve the appropriateness and effectiveness of advocacy efforts to promote an enabling environment that supports effective responses to HIV/AIDS[24] (see also section 3.8 Advocacy), and
- building partnerships and/or engaging in joint research initiatives with research organisations and academic institutions to ensure that research initiatives contribute to improving the evidence base about what is effective in responding to HIV/AIDS.

3.10 Scaling up

What do we mean by 'scaling up'?

The term 'scaling up' is used to encompass different strategies to expand the scope, reach and impact of our responses to HV/AIDS. In the Code we use the term to refer to expanding the geographical or population reach of HIV/AIDS-specific programmes and integrating HIV/AIDS-specific interventions within other health programming, such as sexual and reproductive health and child and maternal health programmes, as well as mainstreaming HIV/AIDS within development and humanitarian programming.

Giving the devastating impact of HIV/AIDS in many developing countries, the need for sustained responses of a sufficient scale to affect the dynamics of the epidemic is abundantly clear. The scaling up of responses needs to be as significant a priority for countries where prevalence is low and where it is still possible to prevent epidemics from spiralling out of control as it is in countries where HIV/AIDS is having a more visible impact.

The challenges associated with scaling up are one of the primary motivations for the development of this Code. While considerable expertise and knowledge exist about what works to prevent HIV transmission and meet the range of needs of PLHA and affected communities, many programmes have yet to become comprehensive in their coverage.[25] There is also much more to be done in mainstreaming HIV/AIDS in order to respond more effectively to the causes and consequences of HIV/AIDS. The good practice principles in this section concerning how to scale up can be more readily applied to existing HIV/AIDS programmes and to integrating HIV/AIDS work into other health and related programming, as efforts to mainstream HIV/AIDS are relatively underdeveloped. Section 4.3 considers mainstreaming HIV/AIDS within development and humanitarian programmes and draws on experience to date to guide these emerging approaches to the HIV/AIDS response.

There is much that can be learned from smaller-scale initiatives that has wider relevance and application. However, scaling up NGO programmes is complex. It is critical to recognise and address the new challenges involved in the process of scaling up.[26] Resources need to be made available in a manner that supports the complexity of the process. Careful planning is needed to determine what programmes are capable of being scaled up, given the nature of the epidemic in a given context.[27] Pressures to meet government and/or donor expectations in order to secure continued resources for scaling up must be balanced with the need to maintain community ownership and a realistic assessment of the capacity of organisations to scale up.

There are numerous different strategies[28] for scaling up, including:

- expanding organisational size and/or scope
- applying cascading and multiplication models, which involve the provision of intensive training to groups who can subsequently provide training to others

- adapting concepts and models so that effective programme approaches can be adapted and replicated
- building practical working partnerships to develop joint initiatives to increase the reach and impact of programming through combined efforts
- catalysing and supporting others by providing technical support
- decentralising services by transferring decision-making and programme coordination from a central location to a more local level, and
- influencing laws and policy that affect the effectiveness of HIV programming.

The strategies employed will vary depending on NGO implementing programmes and whether the organisation concerned is a Supporting NGO (see section 1.6 Who the Code is for). Supporting NGOs are likely to play a role in catalysing and supporting others to scale up programmes. This section provides both good practice principles in scaling up for NGOs generally, as well as outline good practice principles in scaling up that are specific to Supporting NGOs.[29]

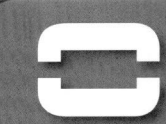

We work to scale up appropriate programmes while ensuring their quality and sustainability.

In determining whether to scale up programmes, we need to ensure that decisions to do so:
- are informed by evidence, including epidemiological, social and behavioural research and programme evaluation findings
- involve PLHA and affected communities in participatory assessment to determine unmet need
- are informed by an assessment of the overall response by the range of organisations and institutions within the particular context, including NGOs and public and private sector agencies, to identify unmet need
- determine which of the strategies for scaling up is most appropriate in the given context, such as whether we are best placed ourselves to address the unmet need, or whether efforts should be directed to advocating for or supporting other organisations or institutions to do so (see section 3.3 Multi-sectoral partnerships)
- build on our particular expertise, strengths and experience, and
- are informed by our ability to acquire the necessary financial and human resources and technical support needed to scale up.

When planning scaling-up strategies, we need to ensure their quality and sustainability by:
- assessing and responding to the implications of scaling up for our organisation (see Organisational capacity in section 3.5)
- building organisational capacity, securing the necessary financial resources and a supportive social and political environment to sustain the programme over time (see section 3.5 Organisational mission and management, and the role of Supporting NGOs below)
- building on the strengths of community initiatives and fostering community ownership of programmes as they are brought to scale
- developing approaches that are sufficiently flexible to address the diversity of need among vulnerable populations, as informed by evidence

- determining an appropriate pace of change, given organisational capacity, level of community mobilisation and time needed to implement scaling up strategies, and
- establishing mechanisms for the collection and analysis of data to enable evaluation of the quality, sustainability and impact of programmes brought to scale (see section 3.6 Programme planning, monitoring and evaluation).

Supporting NGOs need to assist their partner NGOs in scaling up by:
- developing and using transparent criteria for identifying partner NGOs capable of scaling up programmes
- ensuring clarity about, and agreement on, the nature of the scaling up envisaged at the outset
- investing time and money in building capacity to support the scaling up
- allowing and encouraging NGOs to diversify their sources of support
- acknowledging and negotiating tensions among multilateral, government, NGO and donor goals, objectives and strategies for scaling up to ensure that the process of gaining support for scaling up does not undermine the independence of NGOs, and
- actively promoting scaling up as a vital aspect of the global response to HIV/AIDS and facilitating the exchange of information about it among local, national and international stakeholders.

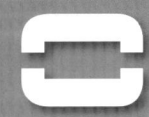 We develop and maintain community ownership and organisational capacity to support scaling up of programmes.

Scaling up activities can have a significant impact on the internal dynamics of an organisation.[30] When planning and implementing scaling up strategies, we need to ensure:
- effective leadership and management of the internal implications of scaling up, including assessment of financial and human resource needs, the appropriateness of our organisational structure, maintenance of organisational cohesiveness and continuity and whether the pace of scaling up is appropriate to our organisational capacity over time
- timely and participatory processes that involve staff and volunteers in designing, implementing, monitoring and evaluating scaling up
- assessment of existing staff and volunteer capacity and provision of appropriate training and development, based on assessed needs
- that staff and volunteers are supported in their work, including in the development of realistic work plans (see section 3.5 Organisational mission and management), and
- that the process of scaling up fosters a learning environment, including building capacity of staff and volunteers to document, reflect upon and analyse their experiences and the experiences of communities about what has and has not worked, to inform organisational development and evaluation of programmes.[31]

The involvement of PLHA and affected communities in the scaling up process and their ownership of programmes are essential to effective scaling up. A particular challenge in scaling up is to balance the need to involve communities and remain responsive to community need while being realistic about the necessary compromises to accountability and quality in order to expand the reach of the programme. When planning and implementing strategies for scaling up, we need to ensure:

- scaling up is built on existing strengths of community initiatives, and community ownership of programmes is sustained as they are bought to scale
- consideration is given to fostering awareness of those in the community whose needs are not being met by existing programmes, particularly those who may be isolated from access to programmes as a result of stigma and discrimination, and
- PLHA and affected communities are involved in the design, implementation and evaluation of scaling up.

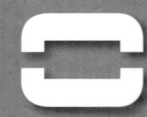 **We monitor and evaluate programmes that are scaled up.**

Expanding the scale-up of existing programmes requires that we are able to monitor and evaluate larger and more complex programmes, often in partnership with other organisations. To do so, we need to ensure that:

- data collection and evaluation methods enable an assessment of focus, coverage, quality, sustainability and impact and are in place before scaling up begins
- quantitative and qualitative indicators are developed and data is collected and used for programme evaluation
- PLHA and affected communities are actively involved in monitoring and evaluation
- organisational capacity is developed to support data collection and analysis
- there is agreement with donors about monitoring and evaluation methods and indicators
- when developing partnership initiatives, there is agreement about monitoring and evaluation methods and indicators, including the use of standardised systems for data collection and analysis, and
- the lessons learnt from scaling up are well documented and experiences are shared both within our organisation and with external partners, promoting a continuing process of improving scaling up efforts (see section 3.6 Programme planning, monitoring and evaluation).

Notes

1   On improving national multi-sectoral responses, see *2004 Report on the Global AIDS Epidemic*, UNAIDS, Chapter 7 and the framework of the 'Three Ones', www.unaids.org

2   DeJong, J., *A Question of Scale? The Challenge of Expanding the Impact of Non-Governmental Organizations' HIV/AIDS Efforts in Developing Countries*, Horizons Program and International HIV/AIDS Alliance, August 2001. See discussion on government-NGO relations in the context of ensuring a coordinated approach to scaling up, pp.42-45, and mainstreaming of HIV/AIDS within the development sector, pp.37-38.

3   In the context of this Code, the constituencies of Supporting NGOs include their NGO partners, such as CBOs, FBOs and organisations of affected communities, including PLHA, sex workers, women's groups and many others.

4   See, for example, the advocacy efforts of the International Federation of Red Cross and Red Crescent Societies: www.ifrc.org and the Masambo fund workplace treatment programme: www.ifrc.org/what/health/hivaids/treatment_masambo.asp

5   See *Working Positively: A Guide for NGOs Managing HIV/AIDS in the Workplace*, UK Consortium on AIDS and International Development, and Holden, S., *Mainstreaming HIV/AIDS in Development and Humanitarian Programmes*, Oxfam, ActionAid and Save the Children, 2004, pp.60-75 (www.oxfam.org.uk) for a discussion of and strategies for 'internal mainstreaming' – i.e. changing organisational policy and practice to reduce susceptibility to HIV infection and the impact of HIV/AIDS on the organisation.

6   Holden, S., ibid., pp.60-75.

7   Ibid. Funding is needed to support human resources and the organisational capacity necessary to reduce an organisation's vulnerability to HIV infection and the impacts of HIV/AIDS. See also Mullin, D. and James, R., *Supporting NGO Partners Affected by HIV/AIDS*, Development in Practice, Vol 14, No. 4, June 2004, 574 585.

8   See *HIV/AIDS NGO/CBO Support Toolkit* (www.aidsalliance.org/ngosupport) and *Raising Funds and Mobilizing Resources for HIV/AIDS Work: A Toolkit to Support NGOs and CBOs*, International HIV/AIDS Alliance 2002. www.aidsalliance.org

9   A wide range of resources is available on the UNAIDS website: www.unaids.org. See also section 5.3 Key resources.

10 See the right to equality and non-discrimination in section 2.4.

11 See Section 2.4 A human rights approach to HIV/AIDS, and Section 3.5 Organisational mission and management.

12 See the right to information in Section 2.4.

13 See the right to privacy in Section 2.4.

14 See section 5.3 Key resources for advocacy tools.

15 See, for example, the Bond Guidance Notes series, including guidance notes on participatory advocacy: www.bond.org.uk

16 See, for example, Watchirs, H., *A Rights Analysis Instrument to Measure Compliance with the International Guidelines on HIV/AIDS and Human Rights*, Australian National Council on AIDS and Related Diseases, 1999. www.ancahrd.org. Legislative audits applying this approach have been undertaken in Nepal and Cambodia. For details see section 5.3 Key resources.

17 For example, partnerships between HIV/AIDS NGOs and organisations working to promote and protect human rights.

18 For example, documenting discrimination and using this information to set advocacy priorities: see section 4.2 HIV/AIDS programming, on stigma and discrimination.

19 Useful resources include: *Advocacy Tools and Guidelines: Promoting Policy Change Manual*, Care International, 2001, www.careusa.org; and the Bond Guidance Notes series on monitoring and evaluating advocacy, www.bond.org.uk

20 Operational research refers to research that is undertaken by NGOs and others in monitoring and evaluating our own programmes. This 'learning by doing' has generated a significant body of knowledge about what works in different contexts, and this must be shared and used to inform our work. See section 3.6 Programme planning, monitoring and evaluation.

21 See, for example, *Joint Advocacy on HIV/AIDS, Treatments, Microbicides and Vaccines*, Canadian HIV/AIDS Legal Network, www.aidslaw.ca

22 See section 2.4 A human rights approach to HIV/AIDS. The right to freedom from torture states that no-one shall be subjected to medical or scientific experimentation without free consent.

23 For example, research such as the Population Council's study on socio-cultural and structural issues likely to affect the introduction of microbicides (www.popcouncil.org) and the need for studies of the long-term consequences of large numbers of orphans in societies and the effectiveness of OVC programmes (*The Framework for the Protection, Care and Support of Orphans and Vulnerable Children Living in a World with HIV and AIDS*, UNICEF, 2004).

24 See, for example, the work of the UNAIDS Global Reference Group on Human Rights and HIV/AIDS, which is working on documenting the evidence for the value of a human rights-based approach in responding to HIV/AIDS. *Public Report: Global Reference Group on Human Rights and HIV/AIDS*, 2003, UNAIDS. www.unaids.org

25 See, for example, *A Question of Scale?, The Challenge of Expanding the Impact of Non-Governmental Organisations' HIV/AIDS Efforts in Developing Countries*, International HIV/AIDS Alliance, 2001, and *Mobilization for HIV Prevention: A Blueprint for Action*, Global HIV Prevention Working Group, 2002. www.kff.org

26 See the discussion of challenges associated with scaling up NGO efforts in *A Question of Scale?*, International HIV/AIDS Alliance, pp.54-60.

27 For example, in low-prevalence countries, with an epidemic that is restricted to specific populations such as injecting drug users, there is likely to be greater cost-effectiveness and impact by scaling up targeted programmes for IDUs, compared with high-prevalence countries where the epidemic is more generalised.

28 Each of these strategies is considered in *Expanding Community Action on HIV/AIDS: NGO/CBO Strategies for Scaling Up*, International HIV/AIDS Alliance, 2000 and *A Question of Scale?*, International HIV/AIDS Alliance, 2001, pp.29-48.

29 The good practice principles in this section draw on the experiences of NGOs in scaling up, examined in detail in the two International HIV/AIDS Alliance publications above. *Expanding Community Action on HIV/AIDS: NGO/CBO Strategies for Scaling Up* provides a practical guide to the process of scaling up.

30 *Expanding Community Action on HIV/AIDS: NGO/CBO Strategies for Scaling Up*, International HIV/AIDS Alliance, p.30.

31 Holden, S., *AIDS on the Agenda: Adapting Development and Humanitarian Programmes to Meet the Challenges of HIV/AIDS*, Oxfam GB, 2003. Chapters 7, 11 and 12 explore experiences in mainstreaming HIV/AIDS internally within the organisation.

Programming Principles

4.1 Introduction

As the devastating impact on individuals, communities and the social and economic development of nations most affected by HIV/AIDS has become increasingly apparent, there is an urgent need to scale up proven strategies, such as targeted HIV prevention programmes and access to antiretroviral therapies (ARVs). However, HIV/AIDS-focused responses alone will not address the inequities that drive HIV infection and worsen the consequences of the pandemic. We must also respond to HIV/AIDS indirectly by addressing developmental factors through a process of mainstreaming HIV/AIDS (see Development in section 2.4).

The term **HIV/AIDS programmes** refers to work such as HIV prevention and treatment, care and support programmes for PLHA, or HIV/AIDS-focused interventions that are integrated within broader health and related programming. The goal of HIV/AIDS programming relates specifically to HIV/AIDS (for example, preventing HIV transmission or reducing HIV-related stigma and discrimination).[1]

The term **mainstreaming HIV/AIDS** refers to adapting development and humanitarian programmes to ensure they address the underlying causes of vulnerability to HIV infection and the consequences of HIV/AIDS. The focus of such programmes, however, remains the original goal (for example, improving household incomes or food security, or raising literacy rates).[2]

This chapter considers both direct and indirect approaches to responding to HIV/AIDS. Section 4.2 provides good practice principles for HIV/AIDS programming, including integrating HIV/AIDS-specific interventions within broader health programming, drawing upon the impressive body of knowledge that exists about how to respond effectively to HIV/AIDS. Section 4.3 considers mainstreaming HIV/AIDS within development and humanitarian programmes. The idea of mainstreaming HIV/AIDS is relatively new, but there is an emerging practice that seeks to strengthen responses to HIV/AIDS by paying particular attention to HIV/AIDS and its consequences in the context of long-term development and humanitarian work.[3] Section 4.3 draws on the available experience to date to guide this process.[4]

HIV/AIDS programming and mainstreaming HIV/AIDS in broader programmes are mutually reinforcing approaches. For example, micro-financing programmes can assist households to increase their income and build assets, both of which can reduce vulnerability to HIV infection and improve capacity to respond to the consequences of HIV/AIDS.[5] Similarly, successful HIV/AIDS programming can reduce vulnerability to HIV infection and stigma and discrimination and maximise access to treatment, care and support, thus facilitating an environment that supports development efforts. Responding to the complexities of HIV/AIDS is best achieved through the combined efforts of NGOs with different areas of expertise doing what each does best, with a heightened understanding of how their work contributes to addressing HIV/AIDS. Different sections of this chapter will be relevant to different kinds of NGOs responding to HIV/AIDS, depending on the nature of their work.

We recognise that the distinction between HIV/AIDS programming and mainstreaming HIV/AIDS is somewhat artificial. For example, humanitarian programming principles for orphans and children made vulnerable by HIV/AIDS (OVC), considered in section 4.3, are often a hybrid of HIV/AIDS and mainstreaming approaches, combining HIV/AIDS-specific interventions, such as HIV/AIDS and sexual health initiatives, with addressing the causes and consequences of HIV/AIDS – for instance, by working to improve access to education. Furthermore, OVC programmes may be stand-alone, or they may be integrated within development programming, or be the product of joint initiatives between HIV/AIDS and development NGOs.[6] Nevertheless, the distinction between the two types of programming is used here to draw out ways in which different NGOs can contribute, and are contributing, to an HIV/AIDS response, both directly and indirectly.

The programming principles set out in this chapter apply to specific kinds of work undertaken by different types of NGO. Therefore the relevance of these good practice principles will depend on the nature of each NGO's work.

The positive interaction between AIDS work and development work

HIV Prevention
- Education about: modes of HIV transmission; means of preventing, or reducing the likelihood of, HIV infection; how HIV differs from AIDS
- Condom promotion and distribution
- STI treatment

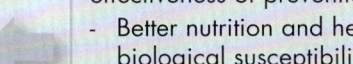

Reduces susceptibility to infection, and increases effectiveness of prevention work:
- Better nutrition and health status ➡ lower biological susceptibility
- Less poverty and livelihoods insecurity ➡ less need to sell sex for survival
- Better health services ➡ greater access to STI treatment and condoms and less iatrogenic infection
- Greater gender equality ➡ women and men more able to act on prevention messages

Reduces numbers of people infected with HIV, and therefore numbers needing care

Education counteracts stigma by challenging misinformation about how HIV is transmitted

Promotes counselling, HIV testing, positive living and seeking treatment. Involvement of HIV+ people may provide role models for this

Care and support to HIV+ people makes AIDS more visible, which counters denial in the general population

Voluntary counselling and testing enables people to discover their HIV status and encourages safer sex practices

Care and support helps HIV+ people to accept their condition and to live positively, including practising safer sex

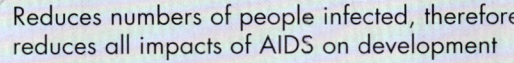

Reduces numbers of people infected, therefore reduces all impacts of AIDS on development

Delayed sexual initiation and use of condoms also affect non-AIDS problems, such as unwanted pregnancies and associated school drop-outs, and STIs

Development
- Poverty alleviation
- Food and livelihoods security
- Health, water and sanitation
- Education
- Humanitarian work following environmental crisis and conflict

Better health services ➡ strengthened systems for provision of counselling, testing, treatment and care for people with AIDS

Less poverty and improved nutrition, water supply and sanitation promote health of HIV+ people

AIDS Care
- Voluntary counselling and HIV testing
- Support for positive living, including material and spiritual support
- Treatment of opportunistic infections
- Antiretroviral treatments
- Care when AIDS develops, at home or in a medical setting

Care and support reduce the impact of illness and death:
- Treatments enable HIV+ people to live and work longer
- Positive living reduces unproductive spending on 'cures', and encourages planning for death, e.g. making a will and arrangements for dependants

From *Mainstreaming HIV/AIDS in Development and Humanitarian Programmes*, Sue Holden, Oxfam Publishing, 2004.

4.2 HIV/AIDS programming

Cross-cutting issues

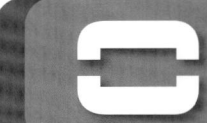 Our HIV/AIDS programmes are integrated to reach and meet the diverse needs of PLHA and affected communities.

The global commitment to providing access to ARVs to the millions of people in the developing world provides new opportunities to improve the effectiveness of the HIV/AIDS response. Maximising access to life-saving drugs will improve the health status of many people living with HIV/AIDS, enhancing their well-being and their capacity to participate in society, and contribute to reducing the stigma associated with HIV/AIDS. It will also provide new incentives for people to find out their HIV status. A massive increase in the provision of voluntary counselling and testing (VCT) and investment in health infrastructure is needed to enable delivery of ARVs.[7] This will provide new opportunities to improve the reach of HIV prevention and improve access to treatment, care and support.

In order to prevent the spread of HIV and respond to the complex effects of HIV/AIDS upon individuals, families and communities, we need to:

- ensure integration between HIV prevention, testing, treatment, care and support programmes within our own organisations, including effective referral pathways
- ensure integration between our programmes and other relevant health and related services and programmes (see also section 4.3 Mainstreaming HIV/AIDS), and
- foster strategic partnerships to facilitate effective referral to other programmes and joint initiatives to meet the diversity of needs of PLHA and affected communities (see section 3.3 Multi-sectoral partnerships).

Given that many people remain unaware of their HIV status, non-HIV/AIDS-specific health services are a vital entry point for the provision of, or referral to, VCT, HIV prevention and HIV/AIDS treatment, care and support programmes (see Voluntary testing and counselling on page 64). Sexual and reproductive health programmes are essential in reducing the risks of HIV transmission and meeting the health needs of both women and men. Preventing and treating sexually transmitted infections (STIs) reduces the risk of people transmitting and acquiring HIV.[8] Integration of programmes and services for family planning, maternal and child health, antenatal care, and prevention and management of STIs and HIV provides a holistic approach to sexual and reproductive health.[9] This is particularly so for women, who are likely to access such services for a range of heath needs but who may not perceive themselves to be at risk of HIV infection, despite the possibility of exposure to HIV through their partner.

People living with HIV are particularly susceptible to tuberculosis, and TB accounts for up to a third of AIDS deaths worldwide.[10] Interventions for TB and HIV prevention and care need to be mutually reinforcing, with joint TB/HIV interventions required to prevent HIV infection, prevent TB, and integrate TB and HIV care for PLHA.

Prevention of Mother to Child Transmission (MTCT) needs to go beyond specific interventions, such as ARVs, counselling on infant feeding[11] and caesarean deliveries, to include HIV and STI prevention among young women and men, quality pre-natal care, access to contraception and counselling about reproductive health options. Effective referral within networks of services enables pregnant women living with HIV/AIDS to have access to VCT services and to HIV treatment, care and support to address their own health needs. A holistic approach to sexual and reproductive health is also likely to meet the range of health needs of sex workers. It is crucial that sexual and reproductive health services are accessible and appropriate for sex workers.

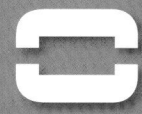 **Our HIV/AIDS programmes raise awareness and build the capacity of communities to respond to HIV/AIDS.**

Our community education and social marketing[12] programmes need to:
- maximise communities' understanding of the consequences of HIV infection
- inform communities about how HIV is and is not transmitted
- increase capacity for risk reduction and risk elimination techniques, including how to access and use prevention commodities
- improve knowledge about and access to VCT, treatment, care and support services
- improve community knowledge about the forms, causes and effects of HIV-related stigma and discrimination
- encourage and support community leadership and community-led initiatives, and
- provide communities with opportunities to participate in addressing HIV/AIDS[13] (see also Addressing stigma and discrimination on page 70).

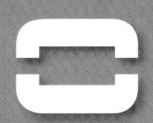 **We advocate for an enabling environment that protects and promotes the rights of PLHA and affected communities and supports effective HIV/AIDS programmes.**

We advocate for:
- review and reform of legislation, such as public health and criminal laws, to ensure that they are appropriately applied to HIV/AIDS and that they are consistent with international human rights obligations[14]
- enacting or improving anti-discrimination and other protective laws and policies, including ethics in research, privacy and informed consent to testing and treatment[15]
- monitoring and enforcement mechanisms, including complaint systems that are appropriate for and accessible to PLHA and affected communities, to guarantee the protection of HIV-related human rights[16]

- establishing or improving legal and related services to enable PLHA and affected communities to know about and enforce their rights[17]
- reform of laws and policy that stigmatise or discriminate against PLHA and affected communities and/or undermine access to information, education and the means of prevention[18]
- review and reform of laws regulating HIV-related goods to ensure widespread availability of prevention commodities[19]
- active political and community leadership on the value and effectiveness of comprehensive harm reduction programmes for people who inject drugs
- reform of health systems to promote application of universal infection control, including safe injection practices and the securing of a safe blood supply
- the development of health service infrastructure to support comprehensive and integrated prevention, testing, treatment, care and support programmes
- wider availability of affordable male and female condoms[20]
- HIV vaccines and microbicide development, including access to community preparedness measures,[21] and
- access to safe, effective and affordable medications,[22] including improved supply of affordable drugs by governments. This also includes international issues regarding compulsory licensing, parallel importing and low international prices for HIV/AIDS-related drugs[23] and national laws relating to regulation of HIV-related goods, to ensure widespread availability of safe and effective medication at affordable prices.[24]

(See also sections 2.4 A human rights approach to HIV/AIDS and 3.8 Advocacy.)

Voluntary counselling and testing (VCT)

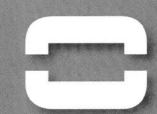

We provide and/or advocate for voluntary counselling and testing services that are accessible and confidential.

In many parts of the world severely affected by HIV/AIDS, as few as one in ten people with HIV know that they are infected.[25] VCT is not only a gateway to treatment, care and support for people living with HIV/AIDS, but also a critical component of HIV prevention.[26]

Increased access to antiretroviral (ARV) therapy is likely to provide new incentives for people to know about their HIV status. It is estimated that by 2005 there will be up to 180 million people in need of VCT annually.[27] There is an urgent need for VCT services on a much larger scale than has occurred to date, including implementing VCT within different types of health settings in order to maximise entry points to HIV prevention and treatment, care and support.[28]

In establishing or scaling up VCT services, we need to provide and/or advocate for VCT services that:

- are voluntary, enabling people to give their informed consent to be tested, based on pre-test information about the purpose of testing and the treatment, care and support available once the result is known
- are confidential, and

- incorporate post-test support and services that advise those who test HIV-positive on the meaning of their diagnosis, and on referral to the treatment, care and support and prevention programmes and services available to assist them. For those who test negative, post-test counselling or discussions offer an important opportunity to reflect on personal risk reduction strategies or to refer people to prevention programmes.

VCT is an important example of the ways in which public health strategies and human rights protection are mutually reinforcing. VCT protects people's rights by ensuring confidentiality, providing information about HIV transmission and personalising discussions of an individual's risk, thus enabling people to make informed decisions about testing and their own risk. In turn, this builds trust between those at risk and the health system, maximising the effectiveness of prevention programmes and ensuring access to treatment, care and support services where necessary. Mandatory testing, on the other hand, engenders fear and erodes trust and co-operation between the individual being tested and the health system, thus undermining prevention efforts.[29]

HIV prevention

There is an impressive body of evidence and experience to guide effective HIV/AIDS prevention. Given that prevention efforts reach fewer than one in five of those at risk, one of the most significant challenges we now face is ensuring that this knowledge is consistently applied in scaling up prevention efforts to reach the millions of people at risk of HIV infection worldwide[30] (see section 3.10 Scaling up).

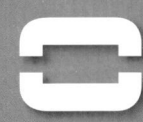 **We provide and/or advocate for comprehensive HIV prevention programmes to meet the variety of needs of individuals and communities.**

Multiple prevention approaches must be employed in combination in order to support individual behaviour change, influence the social norms regarding risk behaviours and address social, economic, legal and policy barriers to effective prevention. Prevention programmes that ensure that the whole spectrum of prevention options is available to those most at risk, including access to and use of condoms and sterile injecting equipment, have been shown to substantially reduce new HIV infection throughout the world.[31]

We need to provide and/or advocate for a comprehensive range of HIV prevention strategies that include:
- accessible and appropriate information about the risks of HIV infection and means of prevention in relation to these risks
- tailored information, education and communication programmes, including sexual health promotion, counselling, discussion groups and peer support
- access to and information about the use of commodities for prevention, including male and female condoms and/or sterile injecting equipment
- social marketing and community education programmes that mobilise communities and influence community norms to support and sustain safer behaviours

- access to voluntary counselling and testing and treatment, care and support programmes, including prevention of MTCT, and
- advocacy efforts to address social, economic, legal and cultural barriers to effective HIV prevention.

There is no evidence that single-focus HIV prevention strategies, such as the provision of condoms alone or abstinence-only approaches, are effective in preventing HIV transmission.[32][33] Single-focus abstinence programmes, particularly for young people, are a response to concerns that comprehensive sexual health and HIV programmes for young people will hasten sexual debut or lead to promiscuity. However, an analysis of research regarding the impact of sexual health and HIV programming on the age of sexual debut of young people and levels of sexual activity does not bear out these concerns.[34] An analysis of national-level survey data from Uganda concluded that among the range of interventions employed in that country – including abstinence, delays in sexual debut, reducing the number of sexual partners and increased condom use – increased abstinence by itself may have made the smallest contribution to lowering the risk of HIV transmission. Interventions had a far greater effect in reducing the number of sexual partners and increasing condom use than they did on the proportion of young people abstaining from sex.[35]

In the context of individual behaviour change, abstinence, fidelity and use of condoms (ABC: *Abstinence Be* Faithful *Condoms*) all have a role to play in reducing HIV transmission. However, it is critical that abstinence and fidelity are not promoted as the preferred approach, with condoms as a last resort, thereby stigmatising condom use. People vulnerable to HIV infection must have access to the full range of prevention options, provided in a manner that is free of judgement, in order for people to be empowered to assess their own risk and make informed decisions about adopting practices appropriate for them. In relation to sexual behaviour, this may include abstaining from sexual activity, reducing the number of sexual partners, delaying commencement of sexual activity, deciding to be faithful to one partner, accessing treatment for STIs and using condoms to prevent HIV and other STIs. In relation to injecting drug use, this may include abstaining from, stopping or reducing drug use, accessing drug treatment, utilising non-injecting methods of drug use and effective use of sterile injecting equipment.

Furthermore the ABC approach, while promoted as a comprehensive approach to HIV prevention, is focused on individual behaviour alone and does not address the societal factors that shape vulnerability. Fidelity requires the agreement of both people in a relationship and does not take into account previous experience or HIV/AIDS status of the individuals involved. Where there is unequal power in sexual relationships, women and girls often do not have the power to negotiate condom use. Sexual violence and coercion, both inside and outside marriage, in peacetime and in conflict, increase the threat of HIV infection for women and girls.[36] This underscores the need for a comprehensive approach to HIV prevention that addresses the underlying causes of vulnerability to HIV and its consequences.

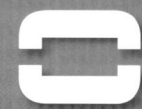 Our HIV prevention programmes enable individuals to develop the skills to protect themselves and/or others from HIV infection.

Information, education and communication (IEC) programmes can comprise a range of approaches, including:
- mass media to inform and establish positive community norms for sustaining safer behaviours for prevention of HIV transmission
- intensive, interactive and personalised counselling, and
- discussion groups and peer support.

We need to address the needs of PLHA and people vulnerable to HIV infection by providing IEC programmes that:
- establish positive community norms for sustaining safer behaviours
- equip people with the necessary understanding and skills to reduce their risk of infection and reduce the risk of transmitting HIV by adopting and sustaining safer sex, safer injecting practices and/or making informed decisions about treatment, birthing and feeding practices to reduce mother-to-child transmission
- provide information, support and strategies to cope with sustaining safer behaviours
- enable discussion of problems and issues people may encounter in sexual and emotional relationships, including the real-life difficulties of sero-discordant relationships, disclosure to sexual partners and the risks of re-infection with different strains of virus where relevant because of the availability of ARV therapies, and
- cover household hygiene and infection precautions.

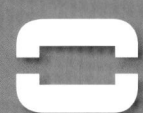 Our HIV prevention programmes ensure that individuals have access to and information about the use of commodities to prevent HIV infection.

Tailored resources and commodities need to be provided for those who cannot afford or access them. These include:
- condoms and lubricant, including choices that exist locally and information on how to use them effectively, and alternatives such as the female condom[37]
- sterile injecting equipment, or in its absence commodities for effective sterilisation, such as bleach, and information on how to use them
- commodities provided through outreach programmes to sites and settings where sexual and drug-taking activity occurs, such as commercial sex premises, non-commercial outdoor sites where people meet to make sexual encounters and places where drug injecting commonly occurs
- commodities provided through a variety of healthcare settings, such as sexual and reproductive health programmes, and
- targeted resources to accompany the distribution of commodities, to ensure their effective use and to promote access to VCT, HIV prevention and treatment, care and support programmes.

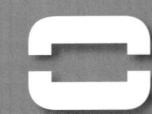 We provide and/or advocate for comprehensive harm reduction programmes for people who inject drugs.

The term **harm reduction** refers to polices and programmes that aim to prevent or reduce the harms associated with injecting drug use.[38]

Injecting drug use is a major factor in epidemics in Asia, North America, Western Europe, parts of Latin America, the Middle East and Northern Africa. In some Eastern European countries, especially the countries of the former Soviet Union, injecting drug use is driving an epidemic among young people.[39] A comprehensive range of harm reduction interventions is essential to effectively address the risks of HIV transmission among people who inject drugs.

We need to provide and/or advocate for comprehensive harm reduction programmes that:

- provide appropriately targeted information preventing HIV transmission, including access to sterile injecting equipment[40]
- provide HIV information, education and communication programmes for people who inject drugs[41]
- provide access to treatment for drug dependence, including substitution treatments such as methadone[42]
- use community outreach strategies to enable people who inject drugs to access HIV prevention information, the means of prevention, drug treatment, VCT and treatment, care and support programmes,[43] and
- address the HIV prevention and treatment, care and support needs of prisoners.[44]

Treatment, care and support

Health systems in the worst-affected countries are often ill-equipped to meet the basic health needs of communities, let alone to provide a comprehensive range of treatment,[45] care and support services for PLHA, their partners, family members and carers. Nonetheless, the global commitment to expand access to ARVs provides new opportunities to advocate for an approach to scaling up that strengthens health systems and builds community capacity. In contexts where health infrastructure is weak and resources are limited, the good practice principles can guide NGOs in advocating for comprehensive and integrated treatment, care and support programmes.

The impact of HIV/AIDS on PLHA, their families, partners, dependants and carers are complex and far-reaching, and include:

- despair about the consequences of progression of the disease, the effects of illness, the possibility of death and the effects of bereavement
- fear of becoming infected or infecting others
- social isolation, including deterioration of family relationships and reduction or loss of social status

- economic implications, including reduction or loss of livelihood or employment, inability to support dependants, pressures on children and young people to provide for or contribute to meeting families' economic and care needs, and
- the many manifestations of stigma and discrimination.

While this section provides good practice principles in HIV/AIDS-related treatment, care and support, the complex consequences of HIV/AIDS on individuals, families and communities underscore the need to foster strategic partnerships to facilitate effective referral to other programmes and joint initiatives to meet the diversity of needs of PLHA and affected communities (see sections 3.3 Multi-sectoral partnerships and 4.3 Mainstreaming HIV/AIDS).

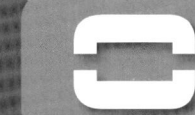 **We provide and/or advocate for comprehensive treatment, care and support programmes.**

Generally, individual NGOs provide only some components of comprehensive treatment, care and support services and programmes, most often home-based care and support programmes, although there are NGOs that provide a wider range of services, including clinical services.

We need to provide and/or advocate for a comprehensive and integrated range of treatment, care and support services and programmes,[46] including:
- accessible and high-quality VCT services (see Voluntary testing and counselling on page 64)
- tailored health information on ARV treatment, including side-effects and adherence issues; treatment for opportunistic infections; and available HIV prevention, care and support services and related health issues, including TB, STI and HIV prevention programmes
- tailored support programmes, including counselling, discussion groups, peer support and spiritual support
- care services, including home-based care, nursing care and palliative care
- HIV treatment programmes, including clinical management of opportunistic infection and HIV-related illness, monitoring and management of disease progression and access to ARV therapy (see also good practice principle in advocating for an enabling environment, including access to treatment, in section 3.8 Advocacy on page 50)
- treatment and prevention of TB and STIs[47]
- support and assistance in relation to non-clinical aspects of treatment, including peer support, adherence and nutritional needs
- information about household hygiene and sterilisation precautions
- a range of support programmes including food, clothing and legal assistance and socio-economic support, and
- support, respite and training for family members and carers of PLHA.

(See also section 4.3 Mainstreaming HIV/AIDS.)

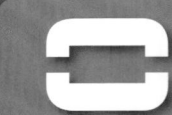 We enable PLHA and affected communities to meet their treatment, care and support needs.

When providing treatment, care and support services for PLHA, we need to:

- involve PLHA, their families, partners, dependants and carers in programme design, implementation and evaluation.[48] This includes the process of building literacy on ARV treatment and HIV health in preparing communities for access to ARV treatment, to ensure that treatment service providers understand community beliefs, knowledge and needs[49]
- provide individual assessment of the treatment, care and support needs of PLHA, taking into consideration the needs of their partners, children, other family members and carers
- provide tailored support programmes that enable people to deal with the consequences of HIV and make informed decisions about their treatment, care and support needs, and
- ensure that the social, economic and psychosocial affects of HIV/AIDS on PLHA, their family and carers are addressed (see Development and humanitarian programmes in section 4.3 on page 76).

An essential part of the response to HIV/AIDS has been, and will continue to be, home- and community-based care. Our care and support programmes need to support partners, other family members, and friends and volunteers providing care and support for PLHA by:

- providing training and resources to ensure carers have appropriate information about HIV/AIDS prevention and care and knowledge of available health services
- supporting carers to develop and maintain the necessary skills to provide quality care, and
- ensuring carers are supported to avoid burn-out, through counselling, peer and social support and respite.

Addressing stigma and discrimination

Stigma is a process of producing and reproducing inequitable power relations, where negative attitudes towards a group of people, on the basis of particular attributes such as their HIV status, gender, sexuality or behaviour, are created and sustained to legitimatise dominant groups in society. **Discrimination** is a manifestation of stigma. Discrimination is any form of arbitrary distinction, exclusion or restriction, whether by action or omission, based on a stigmatised attribute.

HIV-related stigma and discrimination emerge from and reinforce pre-existing gender, race and socio-economic inequities and prejudices about injecting drug use, sex work and men who have sex with men. Pre-existing prejudices and inequities, combined with fears about HIV infection, provide a fertile environment for HIV-related stigma and discrimination to flourish.[50] A significant body of research demonstrates that HIV-related stigma and discrimination is widespread: for example, police harassment of sex workers, injecting drug users and men who have sex with men;

PLHA being refused access to health care; breaches of confidentiality; discrimination in employment; and sexual abuse and violence against women and girls.[51] Families, partners and children of PLHA also frequently bear the burden of stigma and discrimination.[52]

Stigma and discrimination compound vulnerability, and have damaging health, financial, social and emotional consequences for PLHA and affected communities. The effect of stigmatisation and discrimination is to alienate those most affected by HIV/AIDS, making people fearful of knowing their status, adopting preventive measures and accessing counselling, testing, treatment, care and support services.[53] Experience of stigma and discrimination, as well as fear of them, can be internalised, resulting in self-isolation, undermining people's self-esteem, their capacity to sustain safer behaviours and their motivation to exercise control over their own health.[54]

In order to address stigma and discrimination, multiple approaches are needed to ensure that:
- individuals know about their rights, and are supported to respond to stigma, discrimination and their consequences
- communities are supported to examine the nature and impact of stigma and discrimination and play an active role in preventing and eliminating stigma and discrimination
- institutions, such as workplaces and healthcare settings, are supported to promote non-discrimination through effective workplace polices and programmes, and
- laws and policy do not stigmatise PLHA and affected communities.

(See also section 2.4 A human rights approach to HIV/AIDS; section 3.8 Advocacy; and advocating for an enabling environment in Cross-cutting issues for HIV/AIDS programming on page 62).

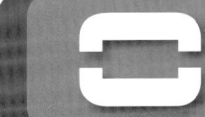

We enable PLHA and affected communities to understand their rights and respond to discrimination and its consequences.

Individuals and communities must be able to name their experience as one of discrimination, understand their rights and have sufficient information and resources in order to take action in response to any discrimination they experience.

We need to provide PLHA and affected communities with:
- easily accessible information about their rights
- advice and support to take action in response to discrimination, through individual advocacy services or effective referral to agencies that can provide them, such as human rights organisations, legal services and unions, and
- support in responding to and addressing the consequences of discrimination, including peer support, counselling, discussion groups and effective referral to housing, employment and related services.

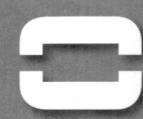

We monitor and respond to systemic discrimination.

Monitoring HIV-related stigma and discrimination, raising awareness about their impact and utilising this knowledge to inform education and advocacy efforts is essential in combating the epidemic. It is important that programmes incorporate a systematic approach to documenting and analysing people's experiences of stigma and discrimination and their efforts to respond to discrimination, in order to understand:

- the nature of stigma and discrimination within a given context, and
- the experiences of individuals and communities of using anti-discrimination complaint mechanisms, other legislatively-based complaint mechanisms and informal strategies for addressing discrimination.

Relevant research, including data derived from monitoring the experiences of stigma and discrimination of PLHA and affected communities, can be used to:

- identify systemic discrimination in particular settings, such as health care, employment, education and prisons
- identify specific institutions that promote stigmatisation of PLHA and affected communities, such as police services, immigration authorities,[55] military services, and the media
- prioritise and inform targeted advocacy and education initiatives in settings where discrimination is common, and
- inform advocacy efforts to reform laws and policies that stigmatise PLHA and affected communities (see advocating for an enabling environment in Cross-cutting issues in HIV/AIDS programming on page 62).

For example, where widespread discrimination in healthcare settings occurs, priority could be given to advocating for the development and implementation of HIV policies and practices that prevent discrimination, including effective procedures to ensure that:

- confidentiality is protected
- testing is voluntary and supported by pre- and post-test counselling
- informed consent is given to testing and treatment
- universal infection control is applied
- staff are trained to support implementation of anti-discrimination policies in practice, and
- complaint mechanisms are available and accessible to address discrimination when it occurs.

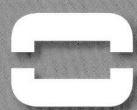

We enable communities to understand and address HIV/AIDS-related stigma.

We need to address stigmatisation of PLHA and affected communities by:[56]
- involving them in the design, delivery and evaluation of programmes designed to address stigma and discrimination
- enhancing community knowledge about the forms, causes and effects of HIV-related stigma and discrimination
- creating opportunities for communities to examine their prejudices and address fears and misconceptions about transmission of HIV
- utilising a range of strategies, including public awareness campaigns, participatory workshop activities and active involvement by communities, in delivery of prevention and care programmes, and
- involving political, religious and community leaders in challenging HIV-related stigma and discrimination.[57]

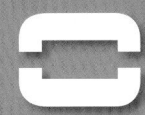

We foster partnerships with human rights institutions, legal services and unions to promote and protect the human rights of PLHA and affected communities.

We need to foster partnerships with human rights organisations and institutions, legal services, lawyers, unions and related advocacy agencies in order to:
- develop awareness of HIV-related stigma and discrimination and encourage the development of HIV-related legal and advocacy expertise
- ensure access to legal advice and advocacy for individuals seeking to enforce their rights
- ensure access to organisations and individuals who can assist in training staff and volunteers on HIV-related legal issues and referral networks, and
- develop joint advocacy strategies and programmes, including among NGOs with human rights expertise and other NGOs responding to HIV/AIDS, to prevent and respond to HIV-related discrimination and stigma and promote the protection of human rights more broadly, including promoting the rights of women and children and addressing the underlying causes of vulnerability, such as poverty and inequities in access to education.

(See also section 3.3 Multi-sectoral partnerships and the good practice principle on advocating for law and policy reform to address the underlying causes of vulnerability to HIV/AIDS on page 83).

4.3 Mainstreaming HIV/AIDS

Section 4.1 defines 'mainstreaming HIV/AIDS' and considers its inter-relationship with HIV/AIDS programming. Mainstreaming HIV/AIDS is a learning process that requires changing attitudes, developing skills and understanding the effects of HIV/AIDS in communities in order to adapt development and humanitarian programming to respond effectively. Mainstreaming requires organisational changes as well as changes to programming. In relation to the organisational changes necessary to support effective mainstreaming, see Chapter 3 – Organisational Principles, particularly Section 3.5 Organisational mission and management; section 3.6 Programme planning, monitoring and evaluation; and Section 3.10 Scaling up. This section focuses on mainstreaming HIV/AIDS in development and humanitarian programmes.

The process of mainstreaming HIV/AIDS

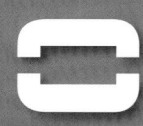

We review our development and humanitarian programmes to assess their relevance to reducing vulnerability to HIV infection and addressing the consequences of HIV/AIDS.

The nature of development and humanitarian work means that all the people with whom we work are likely to be vulnerable to HIV/AIDS and its consequences to some extent. However, a sharper focus on how HIV and AIDS have changed the context for development and humanitarian work is needed, to enable the expertise of development and humanitarian NGOs to be bought to bear in responding to the causes and consequences of HIV/AIDS.

Development and humanitarian NGOs need to explore and understand the way HIV and AIDS affect people's daily lives: in income-generating activities such as agriculture, trading or holding a job; in household activities such as raising children, attending school, caring for family members who are ill, and managing one's own illness; and in how people engage in their communities.[58] The increased burden of illness and caring for those who are sick most often falls on women and girls and older family members, such as grandparents. In turn, this affects people's capacity to participate in the community, rendering them invisible and reducing their access to development and humanitarian programmes. Poverty escalates as the result of illness or death of an income-generating family member. Changes in household composition, such as child-headed, female-headed or grandparent-headed households, may mean that programmes need to be targeted differently or ways of working need to be adjusted in order to reach those who need them and address their particular needs.

Humanitarian NGOs need to understand the nature of vulnerability to HIV infection and the implications of HIV/AIDS in emergency settings. Emergencies involve an array of factors that affect vulnerability to HIV infection and compound the affects of HIV/AIDS:

- poverty and social instability affect the cohesion of families and communities, often weakening social norms that regulate behaviour
- women and children are at increased risk of violence, and can be forced into having sex to gain access to basic needs such as food, water and sanitation
- displacement can bring populations, each with different HIV prevalence levels, into contact with one another
- health infrastructure may be stressed, affecting access to basic care for PLHA and affected communities, and
- poor infection control, lack of availability of condoms and the presence of military forces, peacekeepers or other armed groups can contribute to increased transmission rates.[59]

Mainstreaming HIV/AIDS is a learning process that requires development and humanitarian NGOs to understand:

- how HIV and AIDS change the context for their programming and affect the nature of their work
- whether and how programmes may reduce or inadvertently increase vulnerability,[60] and
- how specific programmes can respond to vulnerability to HIV/AIDS and its impacts, given the particular expertise of NGOs.

Community research is vital to understanding the way in which HIV and AIDS affect people in a given context.[61] We need to involve PLHA and affected communities, including families, partners, dependants and carers of PLHA, in participatory assessment to understand and respond to unmet needs, and in the design, implementation and evaluation of programmes that are adapted to meet identified needs[62] (see sections 3.2 Involvement of PLHA and affected communities and 3.10 Scaling up).

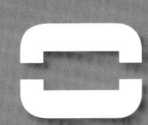

We work in partnerships to maximise the access of PLHA and affected communities to an integrated range of programmes to meet their needs.

We need to focus on our own unique expertise, while working in partnerships with organisations that can address the needs of PLHA and affected communities. Effective referral systems and partnership initiatives between HIV/AIDS programmes and development and humanitarian programmes ensure that PLHA and affected communities have easy access to the range of services and programmes that are appropriate to meet their needs. Measures to address the material and psychosocial needs of PLHA and their families, partners, dependants and carers are also considered in the section on Treatment, care and support in section 4.2 HIV/AIDS programming on page 68 (see also section 3.3 Multi-sectoral partnerships and Cross-cutting issues in section 4.2 on page 62).

Development and humanitarian programmes

Compared with the wealth of knowledge and experience accumulated in HIV/AIDS programming, experience in mainstreaming HIV/AIDS is still relatively limited. Given this, rather than outlining good practice principles informed by evidence, this section draws on experiences to date by providing some examples of how specific kinds of initiative may be adapted to pay particular attention to HIV/AIDS, in the context of long-term development and humanitarian work.[63] These experiences highlight the need to learn by doing, to share experiences and to improve our capacity to monitor and evaluate the effectiveness of our efforts.[64] In turn, this will support advocacy for other sectors to mainstream HIV/AIDS within their core business and the mobilisation of more resources for mainstreaming HIV/AIDS (see sections 3.6 Programme planning, monitoring and evaluation and 3.9 Research).

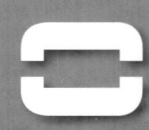 We design or adapt development programmes to reduce vulnerability to HIV infection and meet the needs of PLHA and affected communities.

HIV/AIDS is having a major impact on household **food security, nutrition, and livelihoods**, most visibly in high-prevalence countries. Household food security declines as HIV/AIDS-related illness and death affects agricultural production, transmission of knowledge about farming practices, availability of labour and seasonal employment opportunities for labourers. Food availability decreases through falling production; food access declines due to loss of income; and food utilisation is compromised because of changes in the type and quantity of food consumed. As food consumption declines, malnutrition increases. Malnutrition inhibits immunity to disease and increases the likelihood of opportunistic infections among PLHA.

The need for food can lead to the sale of productive assets, undermining long-term food security; encourage families to withdraw children, especially girls, from school; and result in coping strategies that increase the risk of HIV transmission, notably migration for work and selling sex. The common impact is a decline in income, savings and livelihood opportunities that can increase household and community vulnerability. The impact on individual households depends on a variety of factors, such as economic status, size of the household, which family/members are ill, and the strength of social networks and support.

We need to ensure that development programmes:
- reach households where there are limited employment options, where food supplies are insecure and/or income-generating capacity is affected by HIV/AIDS-related illness or death, and where there is reduced productivity due to increased burden of care, and/or changes in family composition, including grandparent-, women- and child-headed households[65]
- support the capacity of individuals, households and communities to be resilient in the event of ill health, including strategies such as building up protective assets and preserving and investing in family and community relationships[66]

- develop and promote technologies and approaches that address changes in labour and other resources
- facilitate the transfer of traditional and institutional knowledge about life skills and livelihoods across generations
- assess the wider effects of HIV/AIDS, beyond the household, to address the impacts on social systems, human capital, infrastructure, environment and other community assets, and
- track changes in vulnerability over time as households and communities respond and adapt to the impact of HIV/AIDS, and respond accordingly.

Different kinds of development programme can be adapted to respond to the ways that HIV/AIDS has affected the lives of individuals, families and communities. The following are some examples.

Agricultural programmes have a vital role to play in reducing vulnerability to HIV/AIDS and its impacts among rural communities. Several studies have found that agricultural outputs fall by up to 50 per cent in AIDS-affected households, not only decimating earnings, but also leading to a reduction in land under cultivation, the forced sale of productive assets and loss of knowledge as families revert to subsistence crops.[67]

NGOs providing agricultural programmes need to:
- develop and promote labour-saving agricultural technologies
- promote appropriate diversification of crop production, including introduction of new, appropriate technologies that match the labour and nutrition needs of affected households, and
- ensure that PLHA and affected communities have access to appropriate credit, tools and knowledge, such as transfer of customary and institutional knowledge about agricultural practices and skills across generations.

Adjustments to agricultural programmes may include:
- use of threshing machines, mills, wheelbarrows and carts to reduce demands on labour-constrained households
- tools and techniques that are better suited to young, elderly or weak people
- livestock that is better suited to vulnerable households in producing quick returns and aiding accumulation of assets, such as rabbits and chickens, which are easier to look after and reproduce more rapidly
- composting, mulching and applying manure and ashes from the burning of crop residue to increase production, without the use of expensive chemicals[68]
- locating production outside the home, including in kitchen gardens, and intercropping to reduce weeding work.[69]

Micro-finance projects or savings and credit schemes can help households to increase their income and build up assets, so as to reduce their vulnerability to HIV/AIDS and to address its consequences. NGOs providing **micro-finance** and **micro-credit schemes** need to consider how these schemes can be adapted to meet the needs of PLHA and affected communities, without compromising the sustainability of such initiatives. Approaches to doing so may include:
- flexibility in rules governing schemes and allowing for breaks within the savings and credit cycle while retaining membership

- introducing rules to protect the savings of married women, which may otherwise be acquired by their husbands' relatives if they are widowed
- enabling household members to take on responsibility for, or take over, loans if the original member becomes ill or dies, and
- setting up a simple community bank so that people excluded from credit schemes because they are too economically vulnerable can save money and, in time, gain access to the credit facilities of the micro-financing scheme.[70]

The dual challenges of HIV/AIDS and unsafe **water and sanitation** predominantly affect poor and marginalised populations, particularly women and girls and PLHA. Collecting water can make woman and girls vulnerable to sexual violence. Lack of water can force women and girls to exchange sex for access to resources.[71] Water and sanitation issues also affect PLHA, as unsafe water and food often cause diarrhoea, which hastens the progression of HIV-related disease. Access to safe and adequate water is also essential for people taking medicines.

Adjustments to water and sanitation programmes to address access to, and safety of, water for PLHA and affected communities may include:[72]

- establishing a management role in water and sanitation projects for women's groups, particularly widows and other marginalised women, and making them the caretakers of water points, with appropriate incentives for their time
- establishing a safety net to ensure access for the poorest households, who cannot afford to pay for access
- establishing community mobilisation strategies around access to safe water, including addressing misconceptions about contamination of water with HIV and raising awareness among all community members about the rights of PLHA and affected communities, particularly women and girls, and their access to facilities
- establishing mechanisms for reporting and handling complaints regarding access
- placing latrines and water points appropriately to reduce risk of sexual violence
- involving PLHA and women's groups in the promotion of point-of-use safe water treatments
- ensuring safe water strategies and education in all clinic- and community-based HIV/AIDS programmes, including home-based care of PLHA, and
- ensuring safe water and hygiene education in all antenatal care, and that HIV-positive mothers who choose formula feeding have access to safe water.

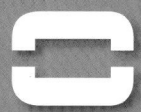 We ensure that our humanitarian programmes reduce vulnerability to HIV infection and address the needs of PLHA and affected communities.

Increasingly, attention is being directed to addressing vulnerability to HIV infection and the effects of HIV/AIDS in emergency settings, including natural crises such as droughts and earthquakes, as well as situations of armed conflict.[73] Humanitarian work in emergency settings has much in common with development work, where programmes address the water and sanitation, food security, housing and healthcare needs of people who are not displaced from their homes.

The Inter-Agency Standing Committee's *Guidelines for HIV/AIDS Interventions in Emergency Settings* (the *Guidelines*) utilise a range of strategies to address vulnerability and the effects of HIV/AIDS, including HIV/AIDS-specific responses such as making condoms available, integrating HIV/AIDS within sexual health and wider primary healthcare programmes, and mainstreaming HIV/AIDS (for example, taking HIV/AIDS into consideration when planning water and sanitation facilities).

The *Guidelines* provide detailed guidance on considering the HIV/AIDS dimensions of emergencies in the preparedness phase, minimum responses in the midst of emergencies, and comprehensive responses in the stabilised phase, in each of the following **sectoral responses**:
- coordination
- assessment and monitoring
- protection
- water and sanitation
- food security and nutrition
- shelter and site planning
- health
- education
- behaviour change communication and information, education and communication (IEC), and
- HIV/AIDS in the workplace.[74]

The extent to which it is possible to mainstream HIV/AIDS in an emergency setting depends upon the stage of the emergency. In the emergency preparedness phase, depending on the different role of NGOs, preparation for an effective response to HIV/AIDS in emergencies should include:
- developing indicators and tools for assessing HIV/AIDS risk and vulnerability in a given context
- including HIV/AIDS in humanitarian action plans and training relief staff on HIV/AIDS, gender and non-discrimination
- protecting and promoting the human rights of PLHA and affected communities, including minimising the risk of sexual violence, exploitation and HIV-related discrimination, and
- planning interventions, developing resources and training staff on the special needs of PLHA and affected communities in each of the areas of sectoral response outlined above.[75]

The *Guidelines* provide **minimum standards** for responses in the midst of emergency and **comprehensive responses** for the stabilised phase of emergencies, in relation to each of the sectoral responses outlined above. Different aspects of each of these responses can be adapted to respond to the ways that HIV/AIDS has affected the lives of individuals, families and communities in emergencies. The following are some examples.

Targeting food aid to HIV/AIDS-affected households is complex, given that the vast majority of people in developing countries are not aware of their HIV status, both because of a lack of availability of testing and fear of testing due to the stigma associated with HIV/AIDS. When providing **food security and nutrition programmes**, food aid needs to reach PLHA and affected communities and the nutritional needs of PLHA need to be addressed. In order to do this, we need to:

- target food-insecure individuals, regardless of their HIV/AIDS status, paying attention to female-, child- and elderly-headed households, families supporting OVC and families caring for chronically ill people
- ensure food aid does not increase stigmatisation when provided to PLHA and affected communities
- plan food baskets that accurately reflect the dietary and nutritional needs of PLHA, including adequate intakes of energy, protein and micronutrients essential to coping with HIV and fighting opportunistic infections, and
- strengthen community capacity to respond to the needs of PLHA and affected communities, including ensuring access to programmes designed to address long-term food insecurity.[76]

Sites in emergencies may take the form of dispersed settlements, mass accommodation in existing shelters or organised camps. When **planning sites and providing shelter**, we need to consider safety and access issues for PLHA and affected communities, including:

- layout of shelters and location of, and access to, facilities that reduce the physical risks for women and girls, such as separate toilet blocks for men and women, and
- layout of shelters and location of, and access to, facilities that address the vulnerability of separated children, especially girls and female-headed households, PLHA and/or those with chronic health conditions.[77]

When providing **health programmes**, NGOs need to integrate HIV prevention and ensure access to basic health care for PLHA and those vulnerable to HIV and its consequences, including:

- ensuring access to basic health care for PLHA and those vulnerable to HIV/AIDS and its consequences
- ensuring a safe blood supply and implementation of universal infection control
- securing condom supplies, together with effective condom distribution and appropriate information for their effective use
- ensuring comprehensive management of STIs, reducing their incidence by preventing transmission through safer sex promotion and treating curable STIs to reduce their prevalence
- ensuring appropriate care for people who inject drugs, including risk reduction information and access to needles and syringes
- ensuring safe and clean delivery of babies, and
- managing the consequences of sexual violence.[78]

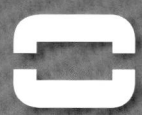 Our programmes for orphans and vulnerable children affected by HIV/AIDS (OVC) are child-centred, family- and community-focused and rights-based.

Why do we use the term 'orphans and children made vulnerable by HIV/AIDS (OVC)'?

Children are affected by HIV/AIDS in a multitude of ways, and not only when a parent dies of AIDS. There are increasing numbers of children living with sick or dying parents. Children are often required to drop out of school to provide care or generate an income for the family. Many children affected by HIV/AIDS are excluded, abused and subjected to stigma and discrimination.

Programmes for orphans and children made vulnerable by HIV/AIDS (OVC) are often a hybrid of both HIV/AIDS and mainstreaming approaches. This section illustrates the use of a human rights approach to programming and the need for partnership approaches that involve different types of expertise in addressing the vulnerability of a particular population group to HIV/AIDS and its consequences (see also sections 2.5 Cross-cutting issues: addressing population vulnerability and 3.3 Multi-sectoral partnerships).

Rights-based approaches to programming for OVC are guided by the principles set out in the Convention on the Rights of the Child (CRC – see Chapter 2). The principles in the CRC include:
- the right to survival, well-being and development
- non-discrimination (see Chapter 2 and section 3.7 Access and equity)
- giving primacy to the best interests of the child in all actions regarding him or her
- fostering participation of children, including the right to express their views freely in all matters affecting them, the right to freedom of expression, and freedom to seek, receive and impart information and ideas of all kinds
- protecting children from all forms of physical or mental violence, injury or abuse, neglect or negligent treatment, maltreatment or exploitation, including sexual abuse, and
- protecting children from economic exploitation and from performing any work that is likely to be hazardous or to interfere with the child's education, or to be harmful to the child's health or physical, mental, spiritual, moral or social development.[79]

OVC programmes need to:
- involve children and young people as active participants
- increase the capacity of children and young people to meet their own needs, through access to quality education, protection from exploitation and developing the skills to care for themselves
- recognise that families and communities are the primary social safety net for OVC and strengthen community-based responses, including engaging leaders in responding to the needs of OVC
- support parents living with HIV/AIDS to fulfil their parenting role, including succession planning for children

- strengthen the caring capacity of families and communities to protect and care for OVC by provision of economic, material and psychosocial support and development of life skills of children, parents and carers (see Treatment, care and support in section 4.2)
- ensure that OVC have access to essential services, including birth registration, schooling, health and nutrition services, safe water and sanitation, and appropriate placement services for those without family or community care[80]
- support children facing stigma and discrimination to cope with and respond to their situation (see Addressing stigma and discrimination in section 4.2)
- pay particular attention to the roles of girls and boys and women and men, including addressing gender roles and norms that affect the vulnerability of women and girls to HIV/AIDS and its consequences
- build and strengthen partnerships with governments, donors, the public sector and the full range of NGOs to coordinate responses, and
- develop responses that are sustainable and capable of replication to meet the long-term needs of OVC.[81]

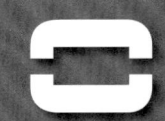

We advocate for an environment that supports effective mainstreaming of HIV/AIDS.

It is critical that global resource mobilisation for the HIV/AIDS response provides additional resources, and that resources are not merely shifted from development work to HIV/AIDS programming or vice versa. Resources for sustainable development initiatives need to be expanded in order to support mainstreaming of HIV/AIDS, just as additional resources are required for HIV/AIDS programming. To bring this about, we need to contribute to creating an environment where there is a common understanding about what mainstreaming HIV/AIDS means and how it can best be achieved.

Given that mainstreaming HIV/AIDS is evolving and evidence of its effectiveness is still limited, it is often difficult to mobilise different sectors to mainstream HIV/AIDS within their core business or raise additional resources to support mainstreaming.[82] However, there are also factors that give impetus to advocating for the need for mainstreaming HIV/AIDS, including:

- a growing recognition that HIV/AIDS work alone does not address the underlying causes of vulnerability to HIV/AIDS and its effects
- the fact that in countries worst affected the impacts of HIV/AIDS are impossible to ignore, and
- recognition that mainstreaming HIV/AIDS draws on the existing expertise and capacity of different sectors that can and should be applied to addressing HIV/AIDS and its impacts through their core business.

We can contribute to creating and sustaining an environment that supports mainstreaming HIV/AIDS by:

- learning by doing, sharing experiences and improving capacity to monitor and evaluate mainstreaming initiatives
- conducting, participating in and/or advocating for research to improve understanding about what is effective

- advocating for governments and private and public sector agencies to mainstream HIV/AIDS within their core business
- advocating for mainstreaming within the HIV/AIDS, humanitarian and development sectors
- advocating for transparency in resource allocation to ensure additional resources are provided for mainstreaming of HIV/AIDS and for specific HIV/AIDS programming, and
- advocating for inclusion of mainstreaming HIV/AIDS within strategic national AIDS frameworks.

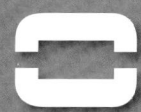 **We advocate for an enabling environment that addresses the underlying causes of vulnerability to HIV/AIDS.**

We need to advocate for review and reform of laws and policy to ensure:
- gender equity for women in accessing credit and income-generating activities and property ownership
- universal birth registration
- protection of the inheritance rights of widows and orphans
- protection of access to land, natural resources, services and credit for PLHA and affected communities
- protection of children against neglect and abuse (physical, sexual and emotional)
- prohibition of exploitative and harmful child labour
- availability and accessibility of social welfare support
- regulation of institutional facilities caring for children, including locating family and community-based care as soon as practicable
- access to education for both girls and boys, especially for girls[83] (see discussion on education below), and
- appropriate placement and guardianship of children who lack adequate adult care.

(See also sections 2.4 A human rights approach to HIV/AIDS and 3.8 Advocacy.)

HIV/AIDS is spreading most rapidly among young women aged 15-24. Improving access to education for girls and boys can make a powerful contribution to reducing vulnerability to HIV infection and the impacts of HIV/AIDS, both directly and indirectly. The UN Millennium Declaration recognises that universal access to primary education and equal access for girls and boys to all levels of education are vital in making the right to development a reality.[84] Literate women are four times more likely than illiterate women to know the main ways to avoid HIV/AIDS.[85] Education also accelerates behaviour change among young men, making them more receptive to prevention messages and more likely to adopt condom use.[86]

NGOs working to improve access to, and quality of, education need to advocate for:
- a diverse range of educational opportunities, including vocational training to enhance income-generating opportunities
- education that enables individuals to develop life skills that will enhance their capacity to reflect on problems, find solutions, make decisions and acquire skills to earn a living
- strategies to ensure that educational environments are non-discriminatory, that they challenge

gender roles and norms and that they encourage changes in attitudes and behaviour that affect the vulnerability of women and girls

- strategies to ensure that educational environments do not expose students to vulnerability to HIV infection, including implementation of policies and procedures for universal infection control and the prevention of sexual exploitation

- strategies to address exclusion from learning of children vulnerable to HIV/AIDS and its impacts, including reducing fees and the cash costs of school attendance, and flexible programming to enable children with competing responsibilities to attend

- creating incentives for school attendance, such as provision of meals

- integration of HIV prevention within the curriculum, including information on sexual health and HIV transmission, and

- effective referral to HIV/AIDS programmes to address the needs of children and young people living with and affected by HIV/AIDS (see section 4.2 HIV/AIDS programming).

Notes

1 In *Mainstreaming HIV/AIDS in Development and Humanitarian Programmes*, (Holden, S., Oxfam, ActionAid and Save the Children, 2004) the author refers to this as 'AIDS work' and 'integrated AIDS work', p.15. See pp.16-17 for a discussion of similarities and differences between AIDS work and mainstreaming HIV/AIDS externally.

2 In the same publication, the author distinguishes between mainstreaming HIV/AIDS internally, which refers to addressing HIV/AIDS within the organisational environment, and mainstreaming HIV/AIDS externally, which refers to adapting programmes. The extent to which mainstreaming HIV/AIDS is applicable where HIV rates are low is considered on pp.40-41. In the Code, the term 'mainstreaming HIV/AIDS' refers to adapting programming (see section 3.5 Organisational mission and management for good practice principles relating to the organisational environment).

3 Ibid., pp.47-49.

4 In particular, section 4.3 draws on a small number of key texts, particularly Holden, S., *Mainstreaming HIV/AIDS in Development and Humanitarian Programmes*.

5 Ibid., pp.81-88.

6 See, for example, Hope for African Children Initiative (HACI), www.hopeforafricanchildren.org

7 *Treating 3 million by 2005: Making it Happen*, WHO, December 2003. www.who.int

8 WHO estimates that over 300 million people are infected each year with curable STIs, a significant proportion of which occur among young people. The presence of such infections during unprotected sex magnifies the risk of HIV transmission by as much as ten-fold. *Report on the Global HIV/AIDS Epidemic 2002*, UNAIDS, p.90.

9 Askew, I. and Berer, M., *The Contribution of Sexual and Reproductive Health Services to the Fights against HIV/AIDS: A Review*, Reproductive Health Matters 2003; 11 (22): pp.51-73. See also the *International Conference on Population and Development (ICPD) Programme of Action*, UN General Assembly, 1994 and *ICPD+5: Key Actions for the Further Implementation of the ICPD Programme of Action*, UN General Assembly, 1999. www.unfpa.org

10 About a third of the 40 million PLHA worldwide at the end of 2001 were co-infected with *Mycobacterium tuberculosis*. For examples of joint TB and HIV interventions, see WHO: www.who.int

11 See *Guidelines on HIV and Infant Feeding*, www.who.int

12 Social marketing is the marketing of public health goods or ideas through traditional marketing channels. See discussion of social marketing of condoms in *Cost Guidelines for HIV/AIDS Prevention Strategies*, UNAIDS, 2000. www.unaids.org

13 *Community Mobilisation and Participatory Approaches: Reviewing Impact and Good Practice for HIV/AIDS Programming*, International HIV/AIDS Alliance, 2004, and *How to Mobilize Communities for Health and Social Change*, Health Communications Partnership.

14 *HIV/AIDS and Human Right: International Guidelines – Revised Guideline 6*, OHCHR and UNAIDS 2002. See Guidelines 3 and 4 www.ohchr.org and *Criminal Law, Public Health and HIV Transmission: A Policy Options Paper*, UNAIDS, June 2002. Search by title, www.unaids.org

15 *HIV/AIDS and Human Right: International Guidelines – Revised Guideline 6*, 2002. See Guidelines 5 and 11.

16 Ibid., Guidelines 5 and 11.

17 Ibid., Guidelines 7 and 8.

18 Ibid., Guidelines 3 – 9.

19 Ibid., Guideline 6.

20 The female condom has been proven effective in reducing the risks of transmission, and surveys indicate that the product would be used more widely by many sexually active women were it more widely available. *Global Mobilization of HIV Prevention: A Blueprint for Action*, Global HIV Prevention Working Group, July 2002, p.14, www.kff.org; WHO, *Evidence for Action on HIV/AIDS and Injecting Drug Use* series).

21 See *Joint Advocacy on HIV/AIDS, Treatments, Microbicides and Vaccines*, www.aidslaw.ca

22 The term 'effective medications' includes ARVs and treatment for opportunistic infections and fixed-dose combinations to support cost-effective delivery and promote adherence, in turn limiting drug resistance. See *Scaling Up Antiretroviral Therapy in Resource-Limited Settings: Treatment Guidelines for a Public Health Approach*, WHO, 2003 revision, p.12 and p.15. www.who.int. Also see Chapter 2, endnotes 17 and 18 for international resolutions useful in advocating access to treatments.

23 See range of resources produced by Médecins Sans Frontières, Access to Essential Medicines Campaign: www.accessmed-msf.org

24 *HIV/AIDS and Human Rights International Guidelines*, Revised Guideline 6.

25 *The Right to Know – New Approaches to HIV Testing and Counselling*, WHO, 2003. www.emro.who.int

26 *Global Mobilization of HIV Prevention: A Blueprint for Action*, p.11. Global HIV Prevention Working Group, 2002.

27 *The Right to Know – New Approaches to HIV Testing and Counselling*, WHO, 2003.

28 See, for example, *Integrating HIV Voluntary Counselling and Testing into Reproductive Health Settings: Stepwise Guidelines for Programme Planners*, Managers and Service Providers, IPPF and UNFPA, 2004. www.ippf.org

29 *The Right to Know – New Approaches to HIV Testing and Counselling*, WHO. For an analysis of the case against mandatory testing, see *Info Sheet 12: Mandatory Testing*, Canadian HIV/AIDS Legal Network, 2000. www.aidslaw.ca

30 *Access to HIV Prevention*, Global HIV Prevention Working Group, May 2003.

31 *Global Mobilization of HIV Prevention: A Blueprint for Action*, pp.8-18, discusses evidence of the effectiveness of combined approaches, including behaviour change, VCT, ARVs, harm reduction programmes and prevention of MTCT. The need for comprehensive prevention programmes is reflected in paragraphs 47-54 of the Declaration of Commitment on HIV/AIDS.

32 *Global Mobilization of HIV Prevention: A Blueprint for Action*, Global HIV Prevention Working Group, p.10.

33 Research indicates that comprehensive programmes are more effective in reducing HIV risk than programmes that promote abstinence alone: Jemmott, J. et al, *Abstinence and Safer Sex: HIV Risk Interventions for African-American Adolescents: A Randomized Controlled Trial*, JAMA 1998, 1529-1536, cited in *Global Mobilization of HIV Prevention: A Blueprint for Action* pp.8-18. See also the Eldis guide, which provides a review of the evidence base in relation to abstinence-only programmes, broad-based sexual health programmes, peer education, mass media HIV awareness and behaviour change, providing summaries of research on the key issues, with links to further sources; www.eldis.org.
The Institute of Medicine, the federal body of experts responsible for advising the United States federal government on issues of medical care, research and education, found that scientific literature, as well as experts who had studied the issue, showed that comprehensive sex and HIV/AIDS education programmes and condom availability programmes could be effective in reducing high-risk sexual behaviours, while no such evidence supported abstinence-only programs (cited in *Ignorance Only: HIV/AIDS, Human Rights And Federally Funded Abstinence-Only Programs In The United States*, Human Rights Watch, September 2002. www.hrw.org).

34 *Dying to Learn: Young People, HIV and the Churches*, Christian Aid, October 2003. www.christian-aid.org.uk

35 Cohen, S., *Beyond Slogans: Lessons From Uganda's Experience With ABC and HIV/AIDS*, December 2003, The Alan Guttmacher Institute, www.guttmacher.org; Singh, S. et al, *A, B and C in Uganda: The Roles of Abstinence, Monogamy and Condom Use in HIV Decline*, December 2003, www.guttmacher.org

36 *2002 Report on the Global HIV/AIDS Epidemic*, UNAIDS, p.65.

37 Research demonstrates that condoms, when used consistently and correctly, are highly effective in preventing transmission of HIV. CDC, National Center for HIV, STD and TB prevention, www.cdc.gov

38 Harm reduction is one of the three complementary approaches to addressing illicit drug use, the others being supply reduction and demand reduction. Supply reduction includes seizing drugs through customs operations, assisting drug producers to grow legal crops and prosecution of drug traffickers. Demand reduction encompasses a range of measures designed to promote a healthy lifestyle free from drugs and to prevent drug use. See *Harm Reduction Principles*, Central and Eastern Europe Harm Reduction Network, www.ceehrn.lt

39 *Report on the Global HIV/AIDS Epidemic 2002*, UNAIDS, p.94.

40 There is compelling evidence that increasing the availability and use of sterile injecting equipment among people who inject drugs contributes substantially to reducing HIV transmission, without contributing to an increase in drug use. *Policy Brief: Provision of Sterile Injecting Equipment to Reduce HIV Transmission*, WHO, 2004, p.2. Early implementation of needle and syringe programmes (NSPs) has been a critical factor in avoiding serious outbreaks of HIV among IDUs. *Global Mobilization of HIV Prevention: A Blueprint for Action*, p.15, Global HIV Prevention Working Group, July 2002.

41 *Effectiveness of HIV Information, Education and Communication Interventions for Injecting Drug Users*, WHO (forthcoming, 2005).

42 Numerous studies demonstrate that substitution treatments reduce drug use, the frequency of injecting and levels of associated risk-taking behaviour. *Policy Brief: Reduction of HIV Transmission Through Drug-Dependence Treatment*, WHO, 2004, p.2. See *Evidence for Action on HIV/AIDS and Injecting Drug Use* series, WHO.

43 *Evidence for Action: Effectiveness of Community-Based Outreach in Preventing HIV/AIDS Among Injecting Drug Users*, WHO, 2004.

44 *Policy Brief: Reduction of HIV Transmission in Prisons*, WHO, 2004. See *Evidence for Action on HIV/AIDS and Injecting Drug Use* series, WHO.

45 'Treatment' includes treatment of opportunistic infections, as well as ARVs.

46 *HIV Care and Support: A Strategic Framework*, Family Health International, June 2001 (www.fhi.org) provides a useful analysis of the components of a comprehensive approach to treatment, care and support.

47 Approximately one-third of PLHA worldwide are co-infected with *M. tuberculosis*, and 70 per cent of them live in sub-Saharan Africa. Tuberculosis is the leading cause of death among HIV-infected people, and HIV has been responsible for a global surge in the number of cases of active tuberculosis. *Report on the Global HIV/AIDS Epidemic 2002*, UNAIDS, p.151.

48 *Policy Briefing No.2: Participation and Empowerment in HIV/AIDS Programming*, International HIV/AIDS Alliance, 2000. www.aidsalliance.org

49 *Improving Access to HIV-Related Treatment*, International HIV/AIDS Alliance; *Antiretroviral Therapy in Primary Health Care: Experience of the Khayelitsha Programme in South Africa*, WHO, 2003, www.who.int

50 *HIV and AIDS-Related Stigmatization, Discrimination and Denial: Forms, Contexts and Determinants*, UNAIDS, 2000. www.unaids.org; and *HIV-Related Stigma and Discrimination: A Conceptual Framework and an Agenda for Action*, Horizons Program, 2002. www.popcouncil.org

51 *AIDS Discrimination in Asia*. Asia Pacific Network of People Living with HIV/AIDS (APN+): www.gnpplus.net; and Human Rights Watch reports, for example: *Policy Paralysis: A Call for Action on HIV/AIDS-Related Human Rights Abuses Against Women and Girls in Africa*, December 2003; *Locked Doors: The Human Rights of People Living with HIV/AIDS in China*, August 2003; *Ravaging the Vulnerable: Abuses Against Persons at High Risk of HIV Infection in Bangladesh*, August 2003; *Just Die Quietly: Domestic Violence and Women's Vulnerability to HIV in Uganda*, August 2003; *Abusing The User: Police Misconduct, Harm Reduction And HIV/AIDS in Vancouver*, May 2003. www.hrw.org

52 See, for example, the role of stigma and discrimination in increasing vulnerability of children and youth infected with and affected by HIV/AIDS, Save the Children (UK), 2001: www.savethechildren.org.uk

53 The effects of discrimination upon vulnerable groups and the consequences for effective responses to HIV/AIDS are examined in the Human Rights Watch reports above and research outlined in *HIV-Related Stigma and Discrimination: A Conceptual Framework and an Agenda for Action*, UNAIDS, 2000, www.unaids.org

54 *Disentangling HIV and AIDS Stigma in Ethiopia, Tanzania and Zambia*, International Centre for Research on Women (ICRW), 2003. www.icrw.org

55 For recommended approaches to travel restrictions, see *Statement on HIV/AIDS-Related Travel Restrictions*, UNAIDS and International Organisation for Migration, June 2004. www.iom.int

56 *Understanding and Challenging HIV Stigma: Toolkit For Action*, Change and ICRW, September 2003. www.changeproject.org

57 For example, *What Religious Leaders Can Do about HIV/AIDS: Action for Young Children and Young People*, UNICEF, UNAIDS and World Council for Religions for Peace, 2003. www.unicef.org

58 *Lessons Learned in Mainstreaming HIV/AIDS, Flyer 5: Researching HIV/AIDS at Local Level* and *Flyer 6: Findings of Local Research on HIV/AIDS*, Oxfam.

59 *Guidelines for HIV/AIDS in Emergency Settings*, Inter-Agency Standing Committee (IASC), 2003, p.6. www.humanitarianinfo.org

60 See discussion of the ways in which development and humanitarian work may actually increase vulnerability to HIV/AIDS and its impacts, Holden, S., *Mainstreaming HIV/AIDS in Development and Humanitarian Programmes*, pp.26-30.

61 Holden, S., *AIDS on the Agenda: Adapting Development and Humanitarian Programmes to Meet the Challenge of HIV/AIDS*, Oxfam GB, December 2003. See practical suggestions for undertaking community research for mainstreaming HIV/AIDS in development work (Unit 7) and humanitarian work (Unit 10).

62 Given that many people are not aware of their HIV status, this is not about seeking to identify people who are living with HIV and AIDS, but rather about using the knowledge within our organisations and communities and our outreach capacity to identify those who are vulnerable to HIV/AIDS and its impacts, e.g. where children are not attending school or where women are no longer involved in community activities or programmes.

63 The examples here are drawn from Holden, S., *Mainstreaming HIV/AIDS in Development and Humanitarian Programmes*, and *Humanitarian Programmes and Guidelines for HIV/AIDS in Emergency Settings*, IASC.

64 *Mainstreaming HIV/AIDS in Development and Humanitarian Programmes*, see discussion on monitoring and evaluation, pp.110-113.

65 See, for example, *Southern Africa... Not Business as Usual*, International Federation of Red Cross and Red Crescent Societies, 2003. This report examines the interface between HIV/AIDS, food insecurity, vulnerability and poverty in Southern Africa and proposes an integrated system of support to households and communities made vulnerable by HIV/AIDS, including home-based care, water and sanitation, food security and income generation, among other features. www.ifrc.org

66 Ibid., see discussion of how households cope with shock and the implications of this for development work, pp.82-84.

67 *Learning to Survive: How Education for All Saves Millions of Young People from HIV/AIDS*, Oxfam, 2004, p.5. www.oxfam.org.uk

68 See, for example, case study on the Natural Farming Network in Zimbabwe, p.42, in Wilkins, M., and Vasani, D., *Mainstreaming HIV/AIDS: Looking Beyond Awareness*, Voluntary Services Overseas (VSO), 2002. www.vso.org.uk

69 *Mainstreaming HIV/AIDS in Development and Humanitarian Programmes*, pp.84-85.

70 Ibid., pp.85-87.

71 Kim, J., *Conceptual Framework: Understanding the Linkages Between Gender Inequity, Lack of Access to Water, and HIV/AIDS*, Rural AIDS and Development Action Research (RADAR), 2004.

72 Ibid., p.21, pp.87-88 and pp.97-99; and *Guidelines for HIV/AIDS Interventions in Emergency Settings*, IASC, including HIV/AIDS consideration in water and sanitation planning, pp.42-43.

73 See *Guidelines for HIV/AIDS Interventions in Emergency Settings*, IASC and The Sphere Project: *Humanitarian Charter and Minimum Standards in Disaster Response*, 2nd Edition, 2004. www.sphereproject.org

74 *Guidelines for HIV/AIDS Interventions in Emergency Settings*, IASC, see matrix on pp.15-19.

75 Ibid.

76 *Guidelines for HIV/AIDS Interventions in Emergency Settings*, IASC, food security and nutrition pp.44-57. See also UN World Food Programme, HIV/AIDS Policy Papers. www.wfp.org

77 *Guidelines for HIV/AIDS Interventions in Emergency Settings*, establishing safely designated sites, pp.58-59.

78 Ibid. Each of these elements is considered in detail, see pp.60–89.

79 As of November 2003, 192 countries had ratified the CRC.

80 *The Framework for the Protection, Care and Support of Orphans and Vulnerable Children Living in a World with HIV and AIDS*, UNICEF, July 2004, www.unicef.org. See discussion of the inadequacies of institutional care in addressing the needs of orphans, p.37.

81 These programming principles and strategies are considered in detail in *The Framework for the Protection, Care and Support of Orphans and Vulnerable Children Living in a World with HIV and AIDS*, UNICEF, and *Building Blocks: Africa-Wide Briefing Notes*, International HIV/AIDS Alliance, January 2003 (www.aidsalliance.org). This series of booklets covers the topics of psychological support, health and nutrition, economic strengthening, education, and social inclusion for communities working with orphans.

82 Holden, S., *Mainstreaming HIV/AIDS in Development and Humanitarian Programmes*, see challenges to mainstreaming, pp.106-113.

83 *Learning to Survive: How Education for All Would Save Millions of Young People from HIV/AIDS*, Oxfam, 2004.

84 Declaration of the UN Millennium Summit, Part III, Development and Poverty Eradication, UN General Assembly 2000 www.un.org

85 Vandemoortele, J. and Delamonica, E., *Education 'Vaccine' against HIV/AIDS*, cited in *Learning to Survive: How Education for All Saves Millions of Young People from HIV/AIDS*, p.2.

86 Ibid.

Appendices

5.1 'Signing on' to the Code

The NGOs that are signatories to this Code have publicly signalled their endorsement of and commitment to the principles it contains, which outline a sectoral vision of good practice in the role of NGOs in responding to HIV/AIDS. Signatory NGOs are provided with a Code logo and may use the strapline *'We endorse the Code of Good Practice for NGOs Responding to HIV/AIDS'* in printed materials and on their websites.

It is not possible to sign on to only parts of the Code. Partial endorsement could undermine the work of other NGO signatories and weaken the collective voice that the Code aims to promote (see section 1.6 About the Code, Scope of implementation).

When the second phase of this project – implementation of the Code – is established, NGOs wishing to sign on to the Code will still be able to do so. An update about this process will be provided on the website of the International Federation of Red Cross and Red Crescent Societies, at www.ifrc.org.

5.2 Implementation of the Code

Scope of implementation

The Code is a comprehensive document that reflects the diverse work of NGOs responding to HIV/AIDS. It is not intended that NGOs commit to implementation of the entire Code. Rather, signatory NGOs will be assisted to implement the guiding and operational principles and those programming principles that are relevant to their work, in a timeframe appropriate to their needs, with an emphasis on continuous improvement over time.

CHAPTER 5

Model for implementing the Code: a work in progress

During consultations with NGOs on the draft Code, a clear theme emerged on the need to provide support to signatory NGOs if they were to implement the Code effectively. In determining a model for implementation, the Steering Committee also drew on the experiences of implementation of other inter-agency codes, namely:

■ *The Code of Conduct for the International Red Cross and Red Crescent Movement and NGOs in Disaster Relief*

■ The Sphere Project: *Humanitarian Charter and Minimum Standards in Disaster Relief,* and

■ People In Aid: *Code of Good Practice in the Management and Support of Aid Personnel.*

Given the diversity of signatory NGOs, the Steering Committee recognised that approaches to using the Code, applying the principles in different contexts and reporting on progress will vary, depending on the type of signatory NGO, such as international NGOs with in-country offices, members of network or federated structures, and national NGOs. Accordingly, the proposed approach to implementation is a flexible one, designed to be refined in collaboration with signatory NGOs.

It is envisaged that signatory NGOs will be assisted to use the Code in their work and to design a process for reporting on strategies for implementing the Code using a process based on *social audit*, including building on monitoring, evaluation and accreditation systems already in place in their organisation.

Social audit is used by not-for-profit organisations and ethical companies to measure and improve performance against social and ethical objectives. There is no 'pass' or 'fail' in a social audit: each organisation can move at its own speed to implement a continuous cycle of improvement. Social audit emphasises institutional learning, as well as training for individuals. It encourages organisations to start from 'where we are', reviewing and building on existing monitoring, evaluation and quality systems when they measure performance. These should be investigated, used and adapted before new ones are introduced.

Once the second phase of the project is established, signatory NGOs will be asked to make a written commitment to implement the Code and to nominate a Code 'champion'. Signatory NGOs will then be entitled to use the strapline *'We are implementing the Code of Good Practice for NGOs Responding to HIV/AIDS'* in printed materials and on their websites.

Supporting implementation

It is envisaged that the Code project will establish a secretariat to support implementation of the Code. The secretariat will provide a focal point for 'marketing' the Code, providing information about it and the process for sign-on and implementation, and helping to network and support signatory NGOs as they use the Code in their work.

The secretariat will map existing mechanisms and support those already available to signatory NGOs, and will identify unmet needs for assistance. Based on this mapping exercise, the secretariat will provide support to signatory NGOs to use the Code in their work, including supporting initiatives for joint activities by signatory NGOs in the same country or region.

It is envisaged that signatory NGOs will apply the Code in different ways – for example, developing training modules with partner NGOs or member organisations, or using the principles contained in the

Code to develop indicators appropriate for the epidemic context within which they work, which can then be used when developing, implementing and evaluating specific programmes. People In Aid and The Sphere Project offer useful examples of possible activities, including workshops, baseline studies, resource centres, pilot programmes and expert advice, that could be provided to signatory NGOs. Many NGOs will already have in place systems of monitoring, evaluation, quality assurance or accreditation. The secretariat will offer signatory NGOs assistance to use existing systems wherever possible to measure their own performance in implementing the Code, including improving accountability.

The Steering Committee has commenced planning for this second phase of the project, including securing the necessary funds. Further information on phase two will be available on the website of the International Federation of Red Cross and Red Crescent Societies.

Electronic version and future revision of the Code

The website of the International Federation of Red Cross and Red Crescent Societies carries an electronic version of the Code, which includes hyperlinks to secondary sources of information, at www.ifrc.org. It is envisaged that the Code will be translated into French, Spanish and Russian as part of the second phase of the project.

The Code is a 'living' document that will need to be revised in order to continue to reflect the principles and practices, and evidence base, that underscore successful NGO responses to HIV/AIDS and provide up-to-date resources to support its implementation. Comments are welcome and a feedback form is provided on page 108.

5.3 Key resources

HIV/AIDS and human rights advocacy

Declaration of Commitment on HIV/AIDS, United Nations General Assembly Special Session on HIV/AIDS (UNGASS), 25-27 June 2001. www.un.org

Advocacy Guide to the Declaration of Commitment on HIV/AIDS, International Council of AIDS Service Organisations (ICASO), October 2001. www.icaso.org

HIV/AIDS and Human Rights: International Guidelines, Office of the United Nations High Commissioner for Human Rights (OHCHR) and the Joint United Nations Programme on HIV/AIDS (UNAIDS), United Nations, New York and Geneva, 1998. The *Guidelines* have been revised to reflect new standards in HIV/AIDS treatment and evolving international law on the right to health. *HIV/AIDS and Human Rights: International Guidelines, Revised Guideline 6, Access to Prevention, Treatment, Care and Support*, OHCHR and UNAIDS, March 2002. Both are available at www.ohchr.org

NGO Summary of the International Guidelines on HIV/AIDS and Human Rights and An Advocate's Guide to International Guidelines on HIV/AIDS and Human Rights, ICASO, 1999. www.icaso.org

Watchirs, H., *A Rights Analysis Instrument to Measure Compliance with the International Guidelines on HIV/AIDS and Human Rights*, Australian National Council on AIDS and Related Diseases, 1999. www.ancahrd.org

Legislative audits applying this approach have been undertaken in Nepal and Cambodia:
- *HIV/AIDS and Human Rights: A Legislative Audit*, National Centre for AIDS and STD Control, POLICY Project Nepal and Forum for Women, Law and Development, 2004.
- Ward, C. and Watchirs, H., *Cambodian HIV/AIDS and Human Rights Legislative Audit*, USAID and POLICY Project Cambodia, 2003. www.policyproject.com

Programming HIV/AIDS: A Human Rights Approach – A Tool for Development and Community-Based Organizations Responding to HIV/AIDS, Canadian HIV/AIDS Legal Network, 2004. www.aidslaw.ca

HIV/AIDS and Human Rights in a Nutshell, ICASO and the International Health and Human Rights Programme of the Francois-Xavier Bagnoud Centre for Health and Human Rights, Harvard School of Public Health, 2004. www. caso.org

Vision Paper: *HIV-Positive Women and Human Rights*, International Community of Women Living with HIV/AIDS (ICW), 2004. www.icw.org

Advocacy Guide for HIV/AIDS, June 2001, and Advocacy Guide to Sexual and Reproductive Health Rights, International Planned Parenthood Federation, July 2001. www.ippf.org

Advocacy in Action – A Toolkit to Support NGOs and CBOs Responding to HIV/AIDS, International HIV/AIDS Alliance, June 2002. www.aidsalliance.org

Advocacy Tools and Guidelines: Promoting Policy Change Manual, Care International, 2001. www.careusa.org

Bringing Rights to Bear: An Advocate's Guide to Work of UN Treaty Monitoring Bodies on Reproductive and Sexual Rights, Center for Reproductive Rights, 2002. www.crlp.org

Fulfilling Reproductive Rights for Women Affected by HIV: A Tool for Monitoring Achievement of Millennium Development Goals, Center for Health and Gender Equity (CHANGE), Ipas, ICW and the Pacific Institute for Women's Health, 2004. www.icw.org

Advocacy Guide: HIV/AIDS Prevention for Injecting Drug Users, International Harm Reduction Association, published by WHO, UNAIDS and UN Office on Drugs and Crime, 2004. www.who.int

Cornwall, A., and Welbourne, A. (Eds), *Realizing Rights: Transforming Approaches to Sexual and Reproductive Well-Being*, Zed Books, London, 2002.

Involvement of PLHA and affected communities

From Principle to Practice: Greater Involvement of People Living with or Affected by HIV/AIDS (GIPA), UNAIDS Best Practice Collection, September 1999. www.unaids.org

Moving Forward: Operationalising GIPA in Vietnam, Care and The POLICY Project, 2003. www.policyproject.com

Vision Paper: *Participation and Policy Making: Our Rights*, International Community of Women Living with HIV/AIDS (ICW), 2004. www.icw.org

Positive Development: Setting Up Self-Help Groups and Advocating for Change. A Manual for People Living with HIV/AIDS, Global Network of People Living with HIV/AIDS (GNP+), 1998. www.gnpplus.net

A Positive Woman's Survival Kit, ICW, www.icw.org

Greater Involvement of PLHA in NGO Service Delivery: Findings from a Four-Country Study, International HIV/AIDS Alliance, summary of the report published by Horizons, July 2002. www.aidsalliance.org

Children's Participation in HIV/AIDS Programming, International HIV/AIDS Alliance, December 2002. www.aidsalliance.org

A Vital Partnership: The Work of GNP+ and the International Federation of Red Cross and Red Crescent Societies, UNAIDS Best Practice Collection, 2003. www.unaid.org

How to Mobilize Communities for Health and Social Change: A Field Guide, Health Communications Partnership, online tool at www.hcpartnership.org

Pathways to Partnerships Toolkit, International HIV/AIDS Alliance, March 1999. www.aidsalliance.org

Building Partnerships: Sustaining and Expanding Community Action on HIV/AIDS, International HIV/AIDS Alliance, March 2000. www.aidsalliance.org

Community Mobilisation and Participatory Approaches: Reviewing Impact and Good Practice for HIV/AIDS Programming, International HIV/AIDS Alliance, forthcoming 2004.

Cross-cutting issues: addressing population vulnerability

As population vulnerability is a cross-cutting issue, resources relevant to working with specific populations can also be found throughout the programming areas outlined in the Key resources section.

The Global Coalition on Women and AIDS, http://womenandaids.unaids.org

Welbourne, A., *Stepping Stones: A Training Package on HIV/AIDS, Gender Issues, Communications and Relationship Skills*, 1995, Strategies for Hope, www.steppingstonesfeedback.org

Gender and HIV/AIDS: Overview Report, www.ids.ac.uk and *Gender and HIV/AIDS: Supporting Resources Collection*, www.ids.ac.uk. Bridge Development and Gender, September 2002.

Integrating Gender into HIV/AIDS Programmes, WHO, 2003. www.who.in

Gendering AIDS: Women, Men, Empowerment, Mobilisation, Voluntary Services Overseas (VSO), October 2003. www.vso.org.uk

Vision Papers: *HIV-Positive Young Women and HIV-Positive Women, Poverty and Gender Inequality*, International Community of Women Living with HIV/AIDS (ICW), 2004. www.icw.org

Men in HIV/AIDS Partnership, POLICY Project, 2003. www.policyproject.com

Working with Men, Responding to AIDS: Gender, Sexuality, and HIV – A Case Study Collection, The International HIV/AIDS Alliance, 2003. www.aidsalliance.org

Rights of Children and Youth Infected and Affected by HIV/AIDS: Trainers' Handbook, Save the Children (UK), 2001. www.savethechildren.org.uk

Children on the Brink: A Joint Report on Orphan Estimates and Program Strategies, UNAIDS, UNICEF and USAID, July 2002. www.unicef.org

Orphans and Other Children Made Vulnerable by HIV/AIDS: Principles and Operational Guidelines for Programming, International Federation of Red Cross and Red Crescent Societies, 2002. www.ifrc.org

Young People and HIV/AIDS: Opportunity in Crisis, UNICEF, UNAIDS and WHO, 2002. www.who.int

Forgotten Families: Older People as Carers of Orphans and Vulnerable Children, International HIV/AIDS Alliance and HelpAge International, 2003. www.aidsalliance.org

What Religious Leaders Can Do about HIV/AIDS: Action for Young Children and Young People, UNICEF, UNAIDS and World Council for Religions for Peace, November 2003. www.unicef.org

HIV/AIDS and Ageing: A Briefing Paper, HelpAge International, May 2003. www.helpage.org

AIDS and Men Who Have Sex with Men, Technical Update, UNAIDS, 2000. www.unaids.org

HIV/AIDS Prevention and Care: A Handbook for the Design and Management of Programs, Chapter 8: Reducing HIV Risk in Sex Workers, Their Clients and Partners, Family Health International (FHI), 2004. www.fhi.org

Sex Workers: Part of the Solution: An Analysis of HIV Prevention Programming to Prevent HIV Transmission During Commercial Sex in Developing Countries, Network of Sex Worker Projects, 2002. www.nswp.org

The Provision of HIV-Related Services to People Who Inject Drugs: A Discussion of Ethical Issues, Canada HIV/AIDS Legal Network, 2002. www.aidslaw.ca

Transgender and HIV: Risks, Prevention, and Care, The International Journal of Trangenderism, 1997. www.symposion.com

Pros and Cons: A Guide to Creating Successful Community-Based HIV/AIDS Programs for Prisoners, Prisoners' HIV/AIDS Support Action Network, 2002. www.pasan.org

Kantor, E., *HIV Transmission and Prevention in Prisons*, HIV InSite Knowledge Base Chapter http://hivinsite.ucsf.edu

Series of 13 Fact Sheets on HIV/AIDS in Prisons, Canada HIV/AIDS Legal Network: www.aidslaw.ca

Population Mobility and AIDS, UNAIDS Technical Update, UNAIDS, 2001. www.unaids.org

Population Mobility and HIV/AIDS, International Organisation for Migration, July 2004. www.iom.int

Keeping Up With the Movement: Preventing HIV Transmission in Migrant Work Settings, The Synergy Project and the University of Washington Centre for Health Education and Research, 2002. www.synergyaids.com

Organisational resources

HIV/AIDS NGO/CBO Support Toolkit, CD-ROM and website, International HIV/AIDS Alliance, 2nd Edition, December 2002. www.aidsalliance.org

Code of Good Practice in Management and Support of Aid Personnel, People in Aid, 2nd Edition, 2003. www.peopleinaid.org

Working Positively: A Guide for NGOs Managing HIV/AIDS in the Workplace, UK Consortium on AIDS and International Development, December 2003. Also provides a good list of resources available online. www.aidsconsortium.org.uk

Developing HIV/Workplace and Medical Benefits Policies – Draft Summary, International HIV/AIDS Alliance, December 2003. www.aidsalliance.org

NGO Capacity Analysis – A Toolkit for Assessing and Building Capacities for High Quality Responses to HIV/AIDS, International HIV/AIDS Alliance, 2004. www.aidsalliance.org

Evaluating Programs for HIV/AIDS Prevention and Care in Developing Countries: A Handbook for Programme Managers and Decision Makers, Family Health International, 2004. Search by title www.fhi.org

UNAIDS resources on programming, monitoring and evaluation: www.unaids.org.

Overseas Development Institute, Research and Policy in Development (RAPID) Framework for Bridging Research and Policy on HIV/AIDS. www.odi.org.uk

Expanding Community Action on HIV/AIDS – NGO/CBO Strategies for Scaling Up, International HIV/AIDS Alliance, June 2001. See Reports and Studies, Scaling up. www.aidsalliance.org

DeJong, J., *A Question of Scale? The Challenge of Expanding the Impact of Non-Governmental Organisations' HIV/AIDS Efforts in Developing Countries*, Horizons Program and International HIV/AIDS Alliance, August 2001.

HIV prevention

Global Mobilization of HIV Prevention: A Blueprint for Action, Global HIV Prevention Working Group, July 2002. www.kff.org

Access to HIV Prevention: Closing the Gap, Global HIV Prevention Working Group, May 2003. www.kff.org

Dying to Learn: Young People, HIV and the Churches, Christian Aid, October 2003. www.christian-aid.org.uk

Best Practices in HIV/AIDS Prevention Collection, Family Health International (FHI) and UNAIDS, 2004. Covers a broad range of topics including mobile populations, emergency relief, prevention and care, and VCT. www.fhi.org

Evidence for Action on HIV/AIDS and Injecting Drug Use Series, WHO, 2004:
- *Policy Brief: Provision of Sterile Injecting Equipment to Reduce HIV Transmission*
- *Policy Brief: Reduction of HIV Transmission Through Drug-Dependence Treatment*
- *Policy Brief: Reduction of HIV Transmission in Prisons*

www.who.int

Evidence for Action: Effectiveness of Community-Based Outreach in Preventing HIV/AIDS among Injecting Drug Users, WHO, 2004. www.who.int

Spreading the Light of Science: Guidelines on Harm Reduction Related to Injecting Drug Use, International Federation of Red Cross and Red Crescent Societies, 2003. www.ifrc.org

Skills Training and Capacity Building in Harm Reduction Work, Open Society Institute (OSI), May 2004. www.soros.org

Unintended Consequences: Drug Polices Fuel HIV Epidemic in Russia and Ukraine, OSI, International Harm Reduction Development, 2003. www.soros.org

UNAIDS resources: search by title at www.unaids.org
- *Partners in Prevention: International Case Studies of Effective Health Promotion Practices in HIV/AIDS*, 1998
- *Sex Work and HIV/AIDS,* June 2002
- *Gender and AIDS: Best Practices/Programmes That Work*, August 2002
- *Prevention of HIV from Mother to Child: Strategic Options*, 1999.

International HIV/AIDS Alliance resources at www.aidsalliance.org
- *An Introduction to Promoting Sexual Health for Men Who Have Sex with Men and Gay Men – A Training Manual*, November 2001
- *Developing HIV/AIDS Work with Drug Users – A Guide to Participatory Assessment and Response*, August 2003
- *Positive Prevention: Prevention Strategies for People with HIV/AIDS*, July 2003
- *Beyond Awareness Raising: Community Lessons about Improving Responses to HIV/AIDS*, July 1998.

Family Health International (FHI) has produced a series of strategic frameworks, including:
Behaviour Change Communication
Sexually Transmitted Infection
www.fhi.org/en
FHI fact sheets offer information on many aspects of HIV prevention, including mobile populations, MSM, MTCT and IDUs: www.fhi.org

Meeting the Behavioural Data Collection Needs of National HIV/AIDS and STD Programmes, IMPACT, FHI and UNAIDS, May 1998. www.fhi.org

Voluntary counselling and testing

The Right to Know – New Approaches to HIV Testing and Counselling, WHO, 2003. www.emro.who.int

Scaling Up HIV Testing and Counselling Services – A Toolkit for Programme Managers, International HIV/AIDS Alliance and WHO, 2004. http://who.arvkit.net

Integrating HIV Voluntary Counselling and Testing into Reproductive Health Settings: Stepwise Guidelines for Programme Planners, Managers and Service Providers, International Planned Parenthood Federation (IPPF) and United Nations Population Fund (UNFPA), 2004. www.ippf.org

Treatment, care and support

The Involvement of People Living with HIV/AIDS in Community-Based Prevention, Care and Support Programmes in Developing Countries, Horizons and the International HIV/AIDS Alliance, July 2003. www.aidsalliance.org

Scaling up Antiretroviral Therapy: Experience in Uganda, WHO, 2003. www.who.int

HIV Care and Support: A Strategic Framework, Family Health International (FHI), June 2001. Search by title, www.fhi.org

Care, Involvement and Action: Mobilising and Supporting Community Responses to HIV/AIDS Care and Support in Developing Countries, International HIV/AIDS Alliance, July 2000. www.aidsalliance.org

Handbook on Access to HIV/AIDS Treatment – A Collection of Information, Tools and Resources for NGOs, CBOs and PLWHA Groups, International HIV/AIDS Alliance, WHO and UNAIDS, 2003. www.aidsalliance.org

Vision Paper: *Access to Care, Treatment and Support*, International Community of Women Living with HIV/AIDS (ICW), 2004. www.icw.org

Community Home-Based Care for People Living with HIV/AIDS, International Federation of Red Cross and Red Crescent Societies, 2003. www.ifrc.org

HIV/AIDS Care and Treatment: A Clinical Course for People Caring for Persons Living with HIV/AIDS, FHI, 2004. Search by title, www.fhi.org

Improving Access to HIV/AIDS-Related Treatment – A Report Sharing Experiences and Lessons Learned International HIV/AIDS Alliance, 2002. www.aidsalliance.org

Improving Access to Care in Developing Countries, UNAIDS, CD-ROM, and *Handbook on Access to HIV/AIDS-Related Treatments: A Collection of Information, Tools and Resources for NGOs, CBOs and PLWHA Groups*, UNAIDS, WHO and International HIV/AIDS Alliance, May 2003. Search by title, www.unaids.org

A Public Health Approach to Antiretroviral Treatment: Overcoming Constraints, WHO, 2003. www.who.int

Breaking Down the Barriers: Lessons on Providing HIV Treatment to Injection Drug Users, Open Society Institute, July 2004. www.soros.org

Saving Mothers, Saving Families: The MTCT-Plus Initiative, WHO 2003. www.who.int

Antiretroviral Therapy in Primary Health Care: Experience of the Khayelitsha Programme in South Africa, WHO, 2003. www.who.int

Gender, AIDS and ARV Therapy: Ensuring that Women Gain Equitable Access to Drugs Within US-Funded Treatment Initiatives, Centre for Health and Gender Equity, February 2004. www.genderhealth.org

Approaches to Caring for OVC: Essential Elements for Quality Service, Institute of Primary Health for UNICEF, February 2001. www.unicef.org

Stigma and discrimination

HIV and AIDS-Related Stigmatization, Discrimination and Denial: Forms, Contexts and Determinants, UNAIDS, June 2000. Search by title, www.unaids.org

HIV-Related Stigma and Discrimination: A Conceptual Framework and an Agenda for Action, Horizons, May 2002. www.popcouncil.org

Disentangling HIV and AIDS Stigma in Ethiopia, Tanzania and Zambia, International Centre for Research on Women (ICRW), 2003. www.icrw.org

Understanding and Challenging HIV Stigma: Toolkit For Action, Center for Health and Gender Equity (CHANGE) and ICRW, September 2003. www.changeproject.org

Protocol for Identification of Discrimination against People Living with HIV/AIDS, UNAIDS, 2000, and *Handbook for Legislators on HIV/AIDS, Human Rights and the Law – Executive Summary*, UNAIDS 1999. Search by title, www.unaids.org/EN

AIDS Discrimination in Asia, Asia Pacific Network of People Living with HIV/AIDS (APN+), 2003. www.gnpplus.net

The ILO Code of Practice on HIV/AIDS and the World of Work, 2001, and *Implementing the ILO Code of Practice on HIV/AIDS and the World of Work: An Education and Training Manual*, 2002, International Labour Organisation. www.ilo.org

The Role of Stigma and Discrimination in Increasing Vulnerability of Children and Youth Infected With and Affected by HIV/AIDS, Save the Children (UK), November 2001. www.savethechildren.org.uk

Men Who Have Sex with Men in Cambodia: HIV/AIDS Vulnerability, Stigma and Discrimination, POLICY Project, 2004. www.policyproject.com

Signs of Hope, Steps for Change, Ecumenical Advocacy Alliance, 2003. CD-ROM multilingual resources, with a particular focus on mobilising and enhancing the role of faith communities and religious leaders in addressing HIV/AIDS-related stigma and discrimination. www.e-alliance.ch

Mainstreaming HIV/AIDS

Holden, S., *Mainstreaming HIV/AIDS in Development and Humanitarian Programmes*, Oxfam, ActionAid and Save the Children, 2004. www.oxfam.org.uk

Holden, S., *AIDS on the Agenda: Adapting Development and Humanitarian Programmes to Meet the Challenge of HIV/AIDS*, Oxfam GB, December 2003. www.oxfam.org.uk

Wilkins, M. and Vasani, D., *Mainstreaming HIV/AIDS: Looking Beyond Awareness*, Voluntary Services Overseas (VSO), 2002. www.vso.org.uk

The Sphere Project: *Humanitarian Charter and Minimum Standards in Disaster Response*, 2nd Edition, 2004. www.sphereproject.org

Guidelines for Interventions in Emergency Settings, Inter-Agency Standing Committee, 2003. www.humanitarianinfo.org

Oxfam resources to support mainstreaming HIV within the work of development and humanitarian organisations: www.oxfam.org.uk

Learning Through Practice: Integrating HIV/AIDS into NGO Programmes: A Guide, POLICY Project and Futures Group, 2002. www.policyproject.com

Mainstreaming Checklist and Tools: Mainstreaming HIV/AIDS into Our Sexual and Reproductive Health and Rights Policies, Plans, Practices and Programmes, International Planned Parenthood Federation (IPPF), 2004. http://content.ippf.org

Multisectoral Responses to HIV/AIDS: A Compendium of Promising Practices from Africa, USAID and Support for Analysis and Research in Africa (SARA), 2003. Resource includes chapters on micro finance, agriculture, capacity development, and working with vulnerable populations such as children, women and refugees. http://sara.aed.org

Building Blocks: Africa-Wide Briefing Notes, International HIV/AIDS Alliance, January 2003. A series of booklets on psychological support, health and nutrition, economic strengthening, education and social inclusion, communities working with orphans, and support to older carers. www.aidsalliance.org

The Framework for the Protection, Care and Support of Orphans and Vulnerable Children Living in a World with HIV and AIDS, UNICEF, July 2004. www.unicef.org

Learning to Survive: How Education for All Saves Millions of Young People from HIV/AIDS, Oxfam, 2004. www.oxfam.org.uk

UN World Food Programme, HIV/AIDS Policy Papers, including *Food Security and HIV/AIDS; WFP's Role in Improving Access to Education for OVC*. www.wfp.org

5.4 Glossary

Acronyms

ABC	Abstinence, Be Faithful, Condoms
ARVs	antiretrovirals
CBOs	community-based organisations
CRC	Convention on the Rights of the Child
FHI	Family Health International
GIPA	the principle of greater involvement of people living with or affected by HIV/AIDS
GNP+	Global Network of People Living with HIV/AIDS
ICASO	International Council of AIDS Service Organisations
ICCPR	International Covenant on Civil and Political Rights
ICESCR	International Covenant on Economic, Social and Cultural Rights
ICRW	International Centre for Research on Women
ICW	International Community of Women Living with HIV/AIDS
IASC	Inter-Agency Standing Committee
IDU	injecting drug use or people who inject drugs
MTCT	mother-to-child transmission
NGOs	non-government organisations
NSPs	needle and syringe programmes
OHCHR	Office of the United Nations High Commissioner for Human Rights
OSI	Open Society Institute
OVC	orphans and children made vulnerable by HIV/AIDS
PLHA	people living with HIV/AIDS
STIs	sexually transmitted infections
UDHR	Declaration of Human Rights (1948)
UNAIDS	Joint United Nations Programme on HIV/AIDS
UNFPA	United Nations Population Fund
UNICEF	United Nations Children Fund
UNRISD	United Nations Research Institute for Social Development
USAID	United States Agency for International Development
VSO	Voluntary Services Overseas
WFP	United Nations World Food Programme
WHO	World Health Organisation

Terminology

Advocacy is a method and a process of influencing decision-makers and public perceptions about an issue of concern, and mobilising community action to achieve social change, including legislative and policy reform, to address the concern.

Affected communities is a term used to encompass the range of people affected by HIV/AIDS, including people at particular risk of HIV infection and those who bear a disproportionate burden of the impact of HIV/AIDS. This will vary from country to country, depending on the nature of the particular epidemic.

Discrimination is a manifestation of stigma (see below). Discrimination is any form of arbitrary distinction, exclusion or restriction, whether by action or omission, based on a stigmatised attribute.

Enabling environment refers to an environment where laws and public policy protect and promote the rights of PLHA and affected communities and support effective programmes.

Harm reduction is used to refer to polices and programmes that aim to prevent or reduce the harms associated with injecting drug use.

HIV/AIDS programmes refers to work that is focused on HIV/AIDS, such as HIV prevention, treatment, care and support programmes for PLHA, or HIV/AIDS-focused interventions that are integrated within broader health and related programming. The goal of HIV/AIDS programming relates specifically to HIV/AIDS (for example, preventing HIV transmission or reducing HIV-related stigma and discrimination).

Mainstreaming HIV/AIDS refers to adapting development and humanitarian programmes to ensure they address the underlying causes of vulnerability to HIV infection and the consequences of HIV/AIDS. The focus of such programmes remains the original goal (for example, improving household incomes or food security, or raising literacy rates).

NGO is used to encompass the wide range of organisations that can be broadly characterised as 'non-government', including Community-Based Organisations (CBOs), Faith-Based Organisations (FBOs) and organisations of affected communities, including people living with HIV/AIDS, sex workers, women's groups and many others, who are active in the HIV/AIDS response.

Scaling up is used to encompass different strategies to expand the scope, reach and impact of our responses to HIV/AIDS. We use the term to refer to expanding the geographical or population reach of HIV/AIDS-specific programmes and integrating HIV/AIDS-specific interventions within other health programming, such as sexual and reproductive health and child and maternal health programmes. We also use it to refer to mainstreaming HIV/AIDS within development and humanitarian programming.

Stigma is a process of producing and reproducing inequitable power relations, where negative attitudes towards a group of people, on the basis of particular attributes such as their HIV status, gender, sexuality or behaviour, are created and sustained to legitimatise dominant groups in society.

Supporting NGO refers to NGOs that provide other NGOs implementing programmes in-country with one or more of the following: technical support; financial support; capacity development and/or advocacy support.

Orphans and children made vulnerable by HIV/AIDS (OVC) We use this term because children are affected by HIV/AIDS in a multitude of ways, and not only when a parent dies of AIDS. There are increasing numbers of children living with sick or dying parents. Children are often required to drop out of school to provide care or to generate an income for the family.

5.5 Acknowledgements

Consultations

The draft *Code of Good Practice for NGOs Responding to HIV/AIDS* was the subject of a wide-ranging consultation process carried out between March–August 2004. Input on the draft Code was provided through face-to-face consultations, e-mail consultations and by written submission. The Steering Committee gratefully acknowledges the efforts of the many organisations and individuals who contributed their expertise to improving the Code.

Project Steering Committee Organisations

- ActionAid International
- CARE USA
- Global Health Council
- Global Network of People Living with HIV/AIDS (GNP+)
- Grupo Pela Vidda
- Hong Kong AIDS Foundation
- International Council of AIDS Service Organisations (ICASO)
- International Federation of Red Cross and Red Crescent Societies
- International Harm Reduction Association
- International HIV/AIDS Alliance
- World Council of Churches

Project host

International Federation of Red Cross and Red Crescent Societies

Project staff

Project Manager and author of the Code: Julia Cabassi (October 2003–December 2004)
Intern: Karen Proudlock (September–October 2004)

Project consultants

Facilitation of consultations: Isobel Mc Connan
Research and recommendations on options for implementing the Code: Sara Davidson.

Funding

The financial and in-kind assistance that has made this project possible is gratefully acknowledged. Financial assistance was provided by: International Federation of Red Cross and Red Crescent Societies, International HIV/AIDS Alliance, Care USA, ActionAid, GNP+, ICASO, the World Council of Churches and the Canadian Red Cross.

In-kind assistance has been provided by: International Federation of Red Cross and Red Crescent Societies, InterAction, HIV/AIDS Alliance Ukraine, Grupo Pela Vidda, Hong Kong AIDS Foundation, World Council of Churches, NGO Forum for Health Geneva, Odyseus, Central and Eastern European Harm Reduction Network, UK Consortium on AIDS and International Development, Canadian Red Cross and Interagency Coalition on AIDS and Development (Canada).

Acknowledgements

Feedback Form

Code of Good Practice for NGOs Responding to HIV/AIDS

All comments submitted will be kept on file at the International Federation of Red Cross and Red Crescent Societies, in anticipation of a revised edition of the Code.

Name: _____

Job title/Organisation: _____

_____

Address: _____

_____

Phone/E-mail: _____

Date: _____

1. What general comments or feedback do you have on any part of the Code? These may include comments on both content and format.

2. What changes do you think would improve the Code? Please be specific and indicate the evidence to support your views.

3. Are there new findings or information that should be reflected in the Code?

4. Are there new key resources that should be included in the Code?

Please send this form to: NGO HIV/AIDS Code of Good Practice Project, Health and Care Department, International Federation of Red Cross and Red Crescent Societies, PO Box 372, 1211 Geneva 19, Switzerland. Fax: +41 22 733 03 95

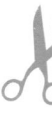